INTERMITTENT FASTING 16/8

Step by Step to Lose Weight, Eat Healthy and Feel Better Following this Lifestyle. Increase Energy and Heal Your Body with Intermittent Fasting. Includes Delicious Recipes

Table of Contents

Introduction

Fasting is something that has been practiced for decades and decades now, starting all the way back to the early days of civilization.

Either for religious, spiritual or health purposes, fasting has been helping individuals since the early days.

You should understand that the core focus of this book is the 16:8 protocol where you are encouraged to eat for 16 hours while keep fasting for 8 hours. [F4]

We chose this particular program because this is essentially the most accessible one of the bunch.

Throughout this book, you will learn about the 16:8 method of intermittent fasting, how it works, and different foods you can use on this method. The book also has amazingly delicious recipes that are easy to prepare.

Intermittent fasting is a health and fitness trend that continues to grow in popularity. People around the world are relying on intermittent fasting to lose weight, improve their overall health and wellbeing, and simplify their lifestyles. This plan has been scientifically proven to improve health when combined with a well-balanced diet.

There are many kinds of intermittent fasting, but this book will cover the 16/8 method specifically. We will explore what it is, why it works, and who it's for. We'll also discuss a step-by-step approach for starting the 16/8 method, whether you are a beginner faster or have been fasting with other methods for a while. We'll investigate how to fast in combination with different diets and whether it should be done. Finally, we'll also cover exercising while fasting and troubleshooting some issues that may come up while fasting.

It's important to note that when using the term "fasting" in this book, we are talking specifically about intermittent fasting, not other kinds. Starting a new fasting program is an exciting time, and we're glad you're reading this book to help you with the process. When you're ready, let's begin!

Chapter 1:
Introducing the 16:8 Intermittent Fasting

What is 16:8 Intermittent Fasting?

On this intermittent fasting method, you fast 16 hours of the day, and only eat during the remaining 8 hours of the day. The fasting window is a total of 16 hours a day; Your fasting window will mostly be during the time you are sleeping. During your fasting window, you will not eat any calories at all. Not eating when your mind and body are accustomed to eating will be difficult, but the challenge is mind over matter, and you matter, so you will succeed. Choose a time to start and stop your feeding window, when the feeding window stops, the fasting window starts, and when the fasting window stops, the feeding window starts, and so on.

How the 16:8 IF diet works

In this method of IF, you only eat within 8 hours and then fast for 16 hours. Most people will think that this will cause them to experience extreme hunger. Normally, we eat all day - from the time we get up in the morning and until we finally go to sleep at night. That will be averaging anywhere from 12 to 14 hours. This is called the fed state.

In this state, the body focuses more on digesting and absorbing recently eaten foods. These processes can take up to several hours. During the fed state, the body's fat-burning processes are at a minimum. It is hard for the body to burn stored fats during the fed state because it relies on the energy derived from recent food consumption.

Insulin levels are high during the fed state. This is a response to the influx of glucose from foods. This more elevated insulin level also hinders fat burning.

After the fed state, the body enters the post-absorptive state. In this state, the body is neither digesting nor processing food. This usually lasts for about 1 to 2 hours after you last ate a meal.

After the post-absorptive state, if you still haven't eaten or drank anything that contains calories, your body enters the fasted state.

During the fasting period, your digestive system does not actively digest solid foods. Instead, it concentrates on fully metabolizing and absorbing the nutrients from foods. This becomes an opportunity to utilize foods fully and turn these into readily usable energy. This energy is quickly used up by the body. Efficient energy use lessens the possibility of converting excess calories into fats.

In the fasted state, levels of insulin are low. The inhibitory effect of insulin on fat-burning is reduced; hence, the body can turn on its fat burning processes at full force. This is why people who go on intermittent fasts burn fats and lose weight without changing their current diet. Even if they still eat the same kinds of foods every day, weight loss is evident.

Steady weight loss is achievable in the 8:16 intermittent fasting diet. This is because the cells burn glycogen stores for energy during the fasted state. When you eat again to break the fast, your body will turn energy into glycogen, instead of turning it into fat cells. This further enhances weight maintenance by reducing the amount of food that gets turned and stored as fats.

One thing that you should know about intermittent fasting is that you can't consider it as a diet plan. In fact, it is an eating pattern, which requires you to schedule your meals to maximize their positive effects on your fitness and health. The pattern involves a cycle composed of separate periods of eating and fasting. So basically, this eating pattern does not require you to change the foods you eat. What you need to change is actually you're eating schedule.

Now, you may be asking yourself if it is really worthwhile to make some changes on when you should eat. The answer is actually a resounding yes.

In fact, IF is an incredible solution if you want to be lean and stay that way without having to follow crazy and difficult diet plans or focus too much on counting calories. In most cases, this eating pattern even requires you to retain your calorie intake when you are still starting out.

In addition, it is a great way of preserving your muscle mass while still keeping your body lean. It is also the simplest strategy if you want to take off unwanted weight and ensure that you stay within your target. You can do that without making excessive changes in your behavior. This makes intermittent fasting simple and doable in the sense that anyone can easily do it while still remaining meaningful as it truly creates a positive difference in your weight and health.

All our lives we heard our parents say, "Breakfast is the most vital meal of the day!", but are they right?

It's an awful tip, suggest the Leangains, the popular 16/8 hour method. With the Leangains, Martin Berkhan introduced the skipping of breakfast, extending the fasting period and taking advantage of the natural fast during sleeping hours. The plan is to fast overnight and the first 6 hours of the day making a total of 16 hours, then eating all your calories in the remaining 8 hours. For example; suppose you woke up at 6 am, waited for the next 6 hours until 12 pm and from 12 pm to 8 pm you get to eat all your carbohydrates and proteins as large, fulfilling meals. You make this way of eating pattern your lifestyle, and the results are obvious.

Why skip breakfast is what you are wondering, right? The idea of 'skipping a morning meal is bad for you' began with studies sponsored by cereal companies to increase sales. This powerful message has been transferred on and has been engraved in the minds of people from so many years that it has become a proper belief. Now imagine... After taking your last meal, you fell asleep, and you woke up to a very low insulin level.

Trust me, the worst thing you can do to yourself right now would be having a high carbohydrate diet which will eventually increase your insulin level, depositing fat stores and shutting the fat burning process for nothing less than 12 hours minimum. Also, this will soon bring the hunger growls in the stomach as the high insulin levels will result in low glucose levels.

Extension of fasting in the 16/8 process does wonders by triggering the metabolic phase, shifting the energy metabolism more on ketones than on glucose. This time-restricted feeding can also decrease the abnormalities linked to obesity. During the 6 hours fast, you can have all the no-calorie liquids, the most important being mineral water. However, the water intake is advised best at certain times. Similarly, snacking is allowed during the fed state, but it's better to have three full meals than nibbling all the time.

Have healthy food with more veggies, fruits, fiber, and protein, but no sugars and no snacking. This will give your body a rest and time to digest the food by breaking it and using it as energy photons to keep you active during the day.

This brings in the significance of exercise or at least staying active in the IMF (InterMittent Fasting) 16/8 . If you cannot go to the gym, do weight lifting exercises such as pushups or squats at home. What matters is that you are not sitting idle. You can go for swimming or to a park for cardio such as jogging or brisk walk. Fasting alone might burn your fat, but it will not help you achieve the desired goal. If we do not use the energy stored in our bodies, then our bodies end up storing this energy as fat, making us lazy. Therefore, exercise is vital for your general wellbeing, health, mental and physical strength and it will also lighten your mood.

No doubt it worked for the bodybuilders, since the IMF 16/8 slows down the muscle tearing process, unlike in other diet programs, thus this is where its fame began. The weight loss encountered by the bodybuilders was tremendous, and the muscle growth was the best part. Many people have the wrong perception that fasting leads to burning muscle instead of burning fat. However, this is not true. Instead, it activates the growth hormone. The hormone in combination with the testosterone burns fat and consequently builds as much muscle as it can. It also keeps us focused and increases our level of alertness.

If you can lose weight, your insulin sensitivities will stay in control, especially in obese men and women, but again why do we need to increase our insulin sensitivity?

Insulin resistance is an omnipresent metabolic problem linked to obesity. Insulin is a peptide hormone secreted by the pancreatic Islets of Langerhans which maintains blood glucose levels. The adipose tissues and muscle insulin really plays an important role in weight loss.

In the muscles, during the fed state, insulin encourages glycogen synthesis through the stimulation of glycogen synthase. To enable energy to be anaerobically released through glycolysis, this activation is necessary, for example, during an intense muscular workout. Muscle cells are not dependent on glucose or glycogen for energy release during the basal state when insulin levels are low. Therefore, low insulin levels divert the attention from burning glucose to finding other sources for energy, and this helps in building muscles as well as weight loss. Low insulin levels also promote the catabolism of protein which is not healthy.

Starvation motivates this breakdown of protein molecules, while a diet routine with intermittent fasting done in the right terms and conditions, does not let the body reach this state.

Getting Started

You should always remember that! Intermittent fasting is not a diet. It is more of a routine than a diet plan, thus once you decide to go for IMF the next step to make is what your fasting and eating time frames will be. Does this mean that you are restricted to a time window? Well, that's where this becomes interesting.

The ideal part is that not only you get to choose the time window yourself, but you can also adjust it according to your comfort zone.

The only thing to be taken care of is that you need to complete your fasting hours. You need to see which meals you are comfortable skipping and how well you'll be able to adjust with skipping them. You can take your routine into consideration with work timings, school timings, etc. This point is like an added bonus to the routine.

Let's check your daily activities to fit in the 16/8 hour time period. Most people prefer starting their fast around bedtime so that half of their fast passes while they are sleeping. They can skip breakfast as part of the fast and have lunch and dinner during their eating window. You follow your time frame according to the routine every day, but what if you are employed and have to work all day, or maybe you are a late-night freak that wakes up late, or you have weekend plans to catch up with your squad?

It's pretty simple! If skipping breakfast isn't an option for you, you can adjust your eating window earlier in the day around 8 a.m. to 4 p.m. If you wake up late, you automatically skip breakfast and keep a night fast. If you have weekend plans such as late-night dinners with friends and family, you straight away shift your fasting window earlier or during the time you are free. These are just examples of how you can adjust your eating window to suit your own eating needs and habits. During your eating window, you must fill yourself up strategically so that you do not get hungry during your fast, and you can even change your eating window every day according to your workload. However, it's best to keep a fixed window and only change it in cases of emergencies, because as a human being our urge for food comes with the daily pattern we set for ourselves and breaking the pattern every day will not only be confusing but will also be inconvenient. Anyways, ensure having a healthy diet.

Appropriate 16/8 Time Frame and Period

The fasting window can be adjusted according to the meal skipping schedule:

skip breakfast: eat lunch and dinner;

skip lunch: eat breakfast in the morning, start your fast, and enjoy dinner;

skip dinner: eat breakfast and lunch and go for an overnight fast

A similar study was conducted at the University of Alabama on a group of men with prediabetes. They also practiced the time-restricted feeding, but at an earlier time frame. The 8-hour period started at 7 am and ended at 3 pm, with all the meals fitting in the time duration. Although there were no signs of weight loss, after 5 weeks both the groups had eye-catching low insulin levels and their insulin sensitivity had also improved amazingly. According to the volunteers, they did not starve although it was tough at the beginning. Later, they noticed a remarkable and controlled decrease in their appetite.

While making sure that your decision of choosing IMF is right, you need to do things accurately. As a beginner, start with baby steps and do not rush yourself. Although the breathtaking results of others might have excited you and you want similar results as soon as possible, just think how they all started. The start must build your stamina rather than breaking it. Learn from the mistakes and experiences of others, even those who dropped out.

"Rome wasn't built in one day, but they worked on it every single day!", and this is how the fasting process operates entirely. A 16-24 hour fast is not a norm for a human being who has to go to work every day, do the chores at their homes, take care of their children, and stay active. We do not advise you to underestimate yourself but give time to your body to adapt to the changes in such a way that it causes no harm physically and mentally. A median American is accustomed to feed their self in a 12-hour cycle, with a 12 hour fast which includes sleeping. This makes them pretty much adapted to the minimum fasting requirement of IMF. Similarly, fasting in many religions have a religious value to people, and therefore they are used to fasting for a month annually.

Considering a person who has never fasted before, it can be tough for them especially looking at other factors such as their age, height, mass, and food preferences. They need to set up a time period to start with.

This will eventually lend the body and cells time to conquer the hunger pangs. The insulin and energy sensitivities will start to store energy for longer periods and to lower insulin to switch from glucose to fat burning. IMF is simple once you get the hang of it, but before you get the hang of it you must go through the tough times.

Make intermittent fasting 16/8 your lifestyle. Once in the zone, and when your body is comfortable with the procedure, "fast more, feed less," and let the words repeat in your mind like a drill to keep the pattern. There is no uncertainty on the fact that the longer the fast, the more effectively it functions and the sooner is the fruit visible, but as we mentioned before, don't be restless. Between trying and triumph, be the "umph" in the triumph! The extended restraining time periods would not harm you, until and unless you are providing your body with what it wants during the eating window. Consistency is going to be of more value than the time frame of your feeding window.

Moving on to how long the drill is preferred to be continued. If you are a beginner, you need to know whether the process goes well with your body, so it is recommended to try the fast weekly or every three weeks, and if you do not face issues of any sort then continue.

Later on, as your two initial weeks are over and you approach the third and fourth week, you start monitoring everything. Adjust your sleep in such a way that you are done eating at least three hours before bedtime. This is because our brain has a nucleus that syncs in our sleeping patterns, dreams, and metabolism through the light that enters our retina. Now we can imagine how late-night browsing on our laptops, iPads, and mobiles, snacking and heavy meals can stray our internal clocks. It also creates confusion between our brain and body since the brain wants to rest and the body full of energy is ready to burn. The best way to stop the functioning of your peripheral clocks is to stop eating at 7 pm.

It is time to tighten up as we enter the fifth and sixth week of time-restricted feeding. You shift the eating window to exactly 8 to 9 hours. By this time, you must have learned to make good food choices. You can continue eating the food that you have been eating, just cut down on the sugar. You could try to incorporate coconut oil in your cooking and add more fish, or fish oil, into your diet. Now is the time where you start shredding your excess fat. The adipose fatty tissue burns, reducing the symptoms of obesity and improving the quality of life.

The eating window describes your lifestyle. Fasting improves your lifestyle to the extent that it reduces the risk of breast cancer in women by 40%. Also, this is irrespective of the food eaten. Isn't it incredible? Further weeks lead to longer fasting and their effects.

Before giving up, glue yourself to it for at least a month, unless you face a medical condition. Do not think of the outcome only in terms of the needle going down the scale. In fact, if the results are positive, the needle on the scale will go up due to muscle buildup, the digestion will get better, and so will you sleep, making you feel good. By the end of the acclimation period, you'll know whether intermittent fasting is a good fit for you or not and whether you can handle it. There's no better teacher than experience.

Good health is an endless journey. As long as we are alive, good health should always remain our goal. However, when we start our journey towards good health, it is always important to set milestones to gauge our progress. Milestones help in judging the progress, and also give us an insight for course correction. Unlike other weight loss measures, intermittent fasting is not linear. It has a wide scope. People practice intermittent fasting for various objectives.

People follow intermittent fasting for 3 main purposes:

1) Losing Weight and Burning Fat

2) Maintaining the Current Weight

3) Holistic Health

You can be practicing intermittent fasting for any of these goals, but you can't judge the progress with the same scale. It is important that you set benchmarks for progress to ensure that the methods are working for you.

Your goals must also be in line with the kind of effort you are putting in. If you are putting in a lot of effort, and yet you are not getting the results, then you would need to do course correction.

Intermittent Fasting for Burning Fat and Losing Weight. This is one of the most popular goals, as people these days are really struggling with weight issues.

There are two ways to judge progress in this area.

1) You should measure the target areas like the waistline, hips, and thighs with a measuring tape to see if the fat burning is taking place.

2) You should weigh yourself on the scale to see if the weight is going down.

There can be anyone of the following scenarios:

1) Your weight is going down, but your waistline remains the same. This happens in the first few weeks of beginning intermittent fasting. Your weight may drop drastically as the body starts dumping a lot of water. You must have patience as the body would start burning fat very soon.

2) You are losing weight as well as your waistline is also going down. This usually happens in the beginning phases, and your body loses weight as well as it burns fat too.

3) Your waistline is going down, but your weight is not going down. This can happen when your body burns fat, but also starts building muscles. The muscles are compact and have more weight. Therefore, you may not see any significant change in your weight on the scale. However, this is a positive thing.

If your observation is something different, then you would need to revisit the whole process and determine the point where you are making a deviation of mistake.

Intermittent Fasting for Weight Maintenance. Maintenance of the existing weight is also a goal people have these days, and it is a very important thing. If the weight starts growing uncontrollably, the day is not far when you will be surrounded by a number of diseases. Therefore, it is important that you get a weight bracket for yourself. You can make changes in your diet and workout routines whenever you notice any significant change in your weight bracket or the waistline.

Intermittent Fasting for Improving Overall Health. Improvement of overall health is a goal everyone must have. If you are healthy, the accumulation of fat is the last thing to happen. Your body is always capable of fighting all the excesses. To judge improvement in health, you will need to take some tests before beginning intermittent fasting, and then keep repeating them at regular intervals.

Best foods to eat during the Eating Window

Intermittent fasting is one of the key solutions for your body to clean out and repair any cellular junk that you have accumulated for several years. This results in the improved function of your body organs and systems. However, you can't expect this eating pattern to perform such an important role successfully if you do not support it with adequate amounts of nutritious foods. The right foods are essential in the process of replenishing and rebuilding your body.

You have to pick whole and good foods with high nutrient density. Eventually, your body will master the art of signaling when it already had enough foods. In return, you will also master the art of listening to your body cues. This will allow you to eat less than what you normally consume before without being too restrictive.

Another thing that you have to remember about intermittent fasting is that it will not work if you follow an extremely restrictive diet. It is because this might cause you to be extremely starved physically and emotionally. This might result in you overeating due to deprivation, so avoid making yourself feel too hungry unnecessarily for a long period.

Just make sure to avoid sticking to processed and unhealthy foods. You still need a well-balanced diet rich in whole and nutritious foods for intermittent fasting to help you in reaching your weight loss and health goals.

How to Follow The 16:8 Method

The 16:8 method is very flexible, and that means you can choose your own specific 8-hour eating window, according to your day. You might work shifts, and that means you sleep at different times. What you should do in that case is pick an 8-hour window which is when you are mostly awake. Obviously!

For example, if you are working nights and you are sleeping between the hours of 10am and 6pm, that means you can eat from 6pm until 2am. You would then probably be working until the following morning when you would head off to sleep, but you could drink coffee (unsweetened and black) to keep you going also, and plenty of water. This might not work for you, so you could think about shifting your pattern and starting it later, perhaps if you don't feel like eating the moment you open your eyes. You could then choose an eating window of 9pm and eat freely until 5am.

It's really up to you!

We've already covered the two main methods most people try with the 16:8, and that is the skipping breakfast and starting to eat at lunchtime routine, or in the case of someone who really needs breakfast because they can't concentrate without it.

It's not only about when you can eat, but it's also about what you eat too. Whilst there are no restrictions and no lists of foods you must eat and foods you shouldn't, always remember that if you suddenly pile a huge breakfast or lunch on your plate after fasting, you're going to end up with stomach ache. That could mean that you end up eating too many calories within your eating window and actually put weight on, or you end up with stomach disturbances for the rest of your eating window, don't get enough fuel during that time because your stomach is so bloated you can't bear to eat, and then you're hungry during your fasting time. It's about choosing carefully, which we'll talk about a little more shortly.

So, how many calories should you eat? It depends on whether you want to lose weight or maintain. A standard calorie amount to maintain weight is 2500 calories per day for a man and 2000 calories per day for a woman. This does depend on the height, current weight, and metabolism of the person, and is really only an average, healthy amount. If you want more solid guidelines on your specific circumstances, speak to your doctor, who will be able to give you a calorie aim plan tailored to your needs.

Within that calorie amount, you should make sure that you get a good, varied diet. That means proteins, carbs, fats, vitamins and minerals. Again, we're going to cover what you can and can't eat, loosely because there are no rules, shortly, but varied is the way to go. Ironically this will also help you enjoy your new lifestyle more, because you're not bored and eating the same things all the time. This is a pitfall many people suffer from regular low-calorie diets; the change is so restrictive that they end up eating the same thing day in, day out, and over time they get so bored and simply rebel against it. This usually ends in a binge day, which causes extreme guilt and then leads them to throw the diet in the bin and go back to eating whatever they want.

Whilst following the 16:8 method, you should also make sure that you drink plenty of water throughout the day, whether fasting or eating. This ensures that you don't become dehydrated and will also aid in digestion. In addition, you should also exercise too!

Now, there are no rules to say that you must exercise whilst following an intermittent fasting routine, but it will help you lose weight faster, and it will help with your general health and wellbeing. Exercise is fantastic on so many levels, not least helping to build lean muscle, which also boosts your ability to burn fat as an energy source. Exercise is also known to help with mental health issues, such as anxiety and depression, as well as stress. We all live stressful lives, and a little exercise can sometimes be enough to reduce it to levels which are extremely manageable. Aside from anything else, exercise can be a sociable and fun activity!

What to eat while fasting and what not to eat

While there are no specific food guidelines as to how you should make up the "Eating" portions of the day, we recommend that you try to stay away from processed food as much as possible and stick to natural alternatives.

Healthy Fats: It is really good for you to consume healthy fats when staying in a clean eating diet. Go for the following

- Olive oil
- Extra Virgin Olive Oil
- Organic Unsalted Butter
- Coconut Oil
- Organic Ghee
- Sunflower Oil
- Avocado

Flours and Grains: Always make sure that you are using 100% whole grain flours that have no additives or preservatives.

- Bread
- Pasta
- Tortillas
- Rice
- Flours
- Soba Noodles
- Cornmeal
- Bread Crumbs

Dairy: Always go for full-fat organic and grass-fed dairy products.

- Plain yogurt
- Buttermilk
- Greek Yogurt
- Sour Cream
- Cream Cheese
- Cottage Cheese
- Milk
- Cheese

Nondairy/Protein Alternative: For protein alternatives, it is good to go for unsweetened plain almond, soy sauce, coconut milk, or even rice.

- Organic Tofu
- Organic Tempeh

Seafood: Sustainable shellfish and fish are the best choices when considering seafood.

Produce: Organic products such as vegetables and fruits are always great for a clean diet.

Meats: When going for meat, it is essential that you go for hormone and antibiotic-free organic meats.

- Poultry
- All-natural bacon
- Uncured deli meats such as ham
- Lean red meats

Salts and Herb: Salts and herbs are self-explanatory. Use them in reasonable amounts.

- Herbs
- Kosher salt or sea salt

Nuts: Nuts as seeds are allowed in a clean diet, so use them liberally

- Unsalted nuts and seeds

- Organic unsalted seed butter/ nut butter

Sweeteners: It is essential that you keep your sugar intake to an as low level as possible, but if your sweet tooth is tingling too much! Then simply go for the following CE approved sweeteners.

- Raw honey
- Date sugar
- Pure maple syrup
- Stevia
- Organic Evaporated cane juice
- Dark chocolate
- Pure vanilla extract
- Unsweetened shredded coconut

Juices: Always go for 100% pure juices!

- Lemon juice (100%)
- 100% fruit juice
- Cold-pressed or homemade 100% vegetable and fruit juices

Thickeners: Some thickeners are allowed in a clean diet such as

- Arrowroot
- Tapioca Starch
- Potato Starch

Canned and Jarred Produce: For canned goods such as tomatoes or beans, only go for the ones that are BPA free.

Condiments: One thing to note while purchasing condiments is to look for the labels. Make sure that they contain no additives, preservatives or sugar. Alternatively, if possible then try to make your own.

- Hot Sauce
- Dijon Mustard
- Reduced Sodium Soy Sauce
- Vinegar

Some additional ingredients: Some more that you should know about:

- Dried berries that are unsweetened
- Liquid smoke naturally crafted
- The chicken broth that is low in sodium
- Agar
- Tomato paste (unsalted)

How to identify processed food

Some precautions to keep in mind

If you think about it on a broader perspective, you would notice that unlike most diets, the only side effect of an intermittent dietary program is that during the early days of your diet, you might feel very hungry.

However, the thing to keep in mind is that hunger often has the tendency to bring general weakness along with it, which in turn might make you feel lethargic to some extent.

You don't have to worry too much about this though as eventually, the feeling of lethargy goes away as your body adjusts itself to the new form of diet.

However, you should keep in mind that if you have any of the following medical condition, you should consult with your physician before embarking on the fasting journey.

- If you have diabetes
- If you are suffering from any kind of blood sugar regulation problem
- If you have low blood pressure
- If you are on regular medication
- If you are underweight
- If you have a history of eating disorders
- If you are female who is trying conceiving
- If you are female with a history of amenorrhea

- If you are a pregnant or nursing mother

Now that everything is pretty much cleared up, below you will find a simple meal plan that is designed to inspire you to make up your own plan.

Now since we are specifically dealing with the 16:8 plan here, the meal plan below is designed in such a manner.

Chapter 2:
Why it is important to maintain healthy weight

You can certainly attain your weight loss objectives by following intermittent fasting along with the keto diet. If you want to speed up the process of weight loss, then here are a couple of simple tips you can use.

Learn to be mindful of the calories you consume. No, you don't have to count every single calorie you consume but learn to make conscious decisions when it comes to food. If you want to lose weight, your body needs to maintain a calorie deficit. A calorie deficit occurs when the energy expenditure of your body is more than the calorie intake. The best way to do this is by following the simple practice of mindful eating. Learn to differentiate between real hunger and hunger triggered by boredom, stress, or any other emotions. Eat only when you are hungry and eat until you are full.

Learn to savor every morsel of food you consume. While eating, ensure that your entire attention is focused on the meal you're eating, and nothing else. Don't be in a rush and don't stuff yourself with food. Instead, set down for a meal, and to your food thoroughly before you swallow it. By chewing your food thoroughly, you're making it easier for your body to digest as well as absorb all the nutrients present in it. It takes your brain about 20 minutes to realize when you are full. If you keep stuffing yourself with food, you will not realize when your tummy is full.

Ensure that you drink plenty of water. Your body needs to stay thoroughly hydrated. Not just to overcome the symptoms of the keto flu, but also to maintain optimal health. You need to drink at least eight glasses of water daily. Always carry a water bottle with you and keep sipping from it regularly. There are plenty of mobile applications; you can use that remind you to drink water regularly.

To tackle hunger pangs, you can drink unsweetened coffee and teas. A cup of herbal tea or green tea is a good idea. Certain enzymes present in green tea help speed up the process of weight loss and increase your body's metabolism. Apart from this, green tea also has a detoxifying effect on your body.

Never leave home, hungry because it increases the chances of eating out will increase. Also, you might not always be able to make healthy food choices on an empty stomach. Always carry a couple of keto-friendly snacks with you. It could be something as simple as a handful of nuts or berries. Whenever you feel hungry, snack on these healthy alternatives instead of reaching for a bag of chips.

While following this diet, ensure that you consume plenty of fatty foods. If you start depriving your body of carbs as well as fats, it will trigger starvation. Don't be scared of fats and load up on healthy fats.

Start adding at least one portion of non-starchy vegetables to all the meals you consume. These foods are not just rich in dietary fibers but are quite nutritious too. Foods like spinach, kale, lettuce, broccoli, and other healthy greens will leave you feeling full for longer. When your tummy is full, it becomes easier to stick to the diet.

Don't forget to do some meal prep. It is quite essential if you want to stick to the diet in the long run. It becomes easy to cook. When all the prep is done beforehand, it could be something as simple as cutting up and portioning all the meats, vegetables, you require in the upcoming week. Maybe you can spend some time and batch cook broths, soups, or even curries. The main idea of meal prep is to reduce the cooking time as much as possible. When all this is done, and everything is in place, you can whip up healthy and nutritious meals within no time.

If you have a sweet tooth, then it might be a little challenging to think about giving up on dessert altogether. However, you don't have to worry.

27

The different recipes given in this book will come in handy. If you want, you can have a handful of berries with some heavy unsweetened whipped cream for dessert. Maybe you can nurse a cup of coffee with some heavy cream in it. Try to avoid sugar as much as possible, and instead, think about healthy alternatives for it. You can make it a friendly ice cream using frozen bananas! There are plenty of other options available, provided you look for it.

Start maintaining a food journal to record the meals you consume. By doing this, you can become quickly conscious of the foods you eat. Apart from this, it is also a great way to keep track of your calorie intake. It comes in handy, especially if you're trying to maintain a calorie deficit. There are different food tracking apps you can use to serve this purpose as well.

Regardless of how hectic your daily schedule is, take some time for some form of exercise or the other. It could be something as simple as talking or even doing yoga at home. As long as you add exercise to your daily routine, you can lose weight. There are only two things you must keep in mind when it comes to weight loss. The first one is to maintain a healthy diet, and the second one is to add exercise.

Before you sit down to eat, drink a glass of water. It helps regulate your appetite and curb any urge to binge. Start using smaller plates while eating. By doing this, you are essentially tricking yourself into eating fewer calories.

Whenever you eat, ensure that you fill yourself up with nutrient-dense foods before you think about eating anything else. There will obviously be instances when you want to eat foods you know you aren't supposed to. Instead of denying yourself these foods, tell yourself you can eat them after you have consumed the necessary fats and proteins.

Try delayed gratification; it works well. Whenever you experience a severe pang to eat something specific that isn't keto-friendly, make a note of it. Have a glass of water and write down all the foods you want to eat. By doing this, you are taking your focus away from these foods. It mostly helps distract your mind.

Whenever you eat out, ensure that you stick to your diet. The general awareness about diets and health has been steadily increasing in recent years. Therefore, wherever you go, you will undoubtedly find some keto-friendly options. If you cannot find any, try customizing a meal for yourself. Maybe you can order two appetizers instead of a starchy main. If you do order a main, add a salad instead of opting for mashed potatoes. It is believed that it takes about 21 days to make or break a habit. Therefore, give your body 21 days to get used to the new diet. In the meanwhile, make a conscious effort to stick to the diet.

If you want to avoid eating out, then maybe you can have a quick snack at home before you head out. Stay away from alcohol if you want to concentrate on losing weight. However, an occasional glass of red wine is perfectly all right.

You can attain your weight loss goals, provided you stick to this diet. It takes patience, commitment, motivation, and resilience. These are certain traits that will come in handy in all aspects of your life. The key to better health lies in your hands!

Chapter 3:
Types of intermittent fasting diets

Fat Fasting Method

The fat loss forever method is an intermittent fasting method in which cheating is allowed. This may be a great thing for people who like to lose weight but cannot stick to some strict diet or the hours of fasting that the other methods require. This method is actually a hybrid method created by Dan Go and John Romaniello, eliminating all the weaknesses that can be faced when practicing other methods. This program is often practiced for twelve weeks, in which one day per week you are allowed to cheat, and right after this day comes the 36 hours of fasting. This last number will scare most of us, right? The creators of this method suggest performing the fasting on the busiest days of the week, so we won't have a lot of time to think of food.

In addition to this method, there is a training program that can aid in gaining muscle and losing even more weight. Many people may find this method difficult, especially those who are not accustomed to fasting. The cheat days could be threatening to some in the sense that during these days they could consume much more food than they normally would. But everything is in the self-control, isn't it?

The 16:8 Method

There are different ways to learn IF. However, they all have the same meaning; all are in seasonal feeding and fasting.

The time to fast – it depends on the time length in different methods. During this time, you have not eaten at all or zero-calorie drinks.

Feeding time – also varies with the length of time in each method. During this time, you can eat whatever you want moderately to avoid too many drinks. It is advisable to eat normally and do not look like compensation during your lack of food. Some features like Warrior Diet may require you to eat foods in a particular way.

As the name implies, this method is divided into two periods; for 16 hours of fasting and 8 hours of feeding time. It is important to monitor your feeding time regularly. This means that you cannot decide to eat from 8 am to 4 pm today and change from 8 pm to 4 am the next day. This is designed to create a schedule that is easy for your body to adapt to and easy to follow. Remember, the hungry hormones are released concerning eating habits? Changing your routine regularly will make you hungry all the time and experience a problem with these hormones.

This method is said to be durable and easy to stick to as you are not required to live without food for a long time, and can easily adapt to the lives of most people in everyday life. For example, the average person sleeps for eight hours. You only need to fast for an additional 8 hours while you are awake, making the fasting period shorter.

For example, if your last meal was at 10 pm, you would fast until 2 pm the next day, and some would sleep, while others would be busy - you won't know exactly when. This method is popular as you can still have dinner with your family or friends before your feeding window closes. Important note: Some research suggests eating late at night produces higher insulin than daytime affects sleep quality and enhances nighttime storage.

Alternate day fasting

This may seem comparable to the 5:2 regiment of fasting, but it is not. It involves fasting daily. You can follow this technique until you lose as much weight as you want, then you can decrease the days of fasting. It allows weight loss to be maintained.

You can move between intermittent fasting units, as daily occurrences are not always constant. Intermittent fasting is not all about pursuing a time-limiting eating window, other parts to it, some are discussed above. Intermittent fasting is flexible, so you can move your eating and fasting time to suit you, but do not keep on changing them continuously; this reduces the impact of fasting on your body.

You can even merge some fasting regiments like the 5:2 method and the 24 hours fast by eating dinner at a certain time before your day of fasting and eating only dinner at the fasting dinner and doing the same for the next day of fasting. With this, you have not been able to consume any calories for twenty-four hours and set your days of fasting as in the 5:2 technique of fasting. Choose the technique and a day of fasting that operates well with you and can readily synchronize with your lives.

A timetable enables you to develop a routine after frequent fasting that will render it simpler to integrate into your lives. It is possible for you to plan but if you cannot, there is no issue. Even if you cannot schedule fasting, you should be open-minded to fasting possibilities. You can fast on a monthly or even yearly basis. Frankly, if you want to lose weight, then annual fasts will not assist you. What such a fasting timetable can assist you with is to offer you time to rest, meditate and reflect on your lives. Several religions and cultures all over the globe do this.

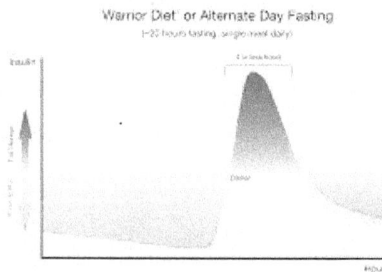

Warrior Diet or Alternate Day Fasting
(~20 hours fasting, single meal daily)

The long-term fasts are usually medically supervised. Fasting for very long periods can be very dangerous thus, medical support is mandatory. Fasting is cumulative, thus if you fast for only two days a week for one year, you will have fasted for one hundred and four days. You do not have to put yourself through extreme fasts constantly, as the benefits will almost be similar. Just try it out, do not seek advice from a friend who lacks adequate information on it, as they will most likely discourage you.

Even as intermittent fasting is great, individuals with diabetes and those receiving medicine may be at danger from lengthy, fast phases. If you do not feel fine, you should stop fasting; being ill is not a component of fasting; only hunger is permitted. If you are on any medication, particularly diabetes medication, a doctor should supervise you during fasting. Before beginning a fasting regimen or nutritional modifications, it is also essential to consult a doctor. Blood glucose is lowered during longer fast due to reduced food intake thus taking the regular dose of medication as you would if you were not fasting; you are at risk of becoming hypoglycemic.

Hypoglycemia has several symptoms like sweating, general body weakness, shakiness, tremors, confusion, and hunger. It may even lead to seizures, loss of consciousness and even death, it is very dangerous. Your blood sugar and medications must be in a state of equilibrium to avoid low or high blood sugar. You can attain this balance with the help of a physician. To avoid hypoglycemia, diabetic medications and insulin must be reduced on the day of fasting.

Intermittent fasting plan

The beauty of social media is that ideas can be shared around the world and gain popularity very quickly. It's probably why you're here, reading this book. On social media you can find many influencers and celebrities who have tried intermittent fasting, and wholeheartedly advocate for it. Whether you want to look like the actors who play superheroes or whether you just want to get healthier, intermittent fasting can help you achieve your goals.

In the introduction, we covered how fasting was used throughout history for health, political, religious reasons. Some of these fasts are very similar to intermittent fasting. In general, intermittent fasting is when you time your eating to fit within a specific window during your day or week. Your fasting hours might just be during the night, or they might extend to a full 24 hours. When comparing intermittent fasting to religious fasting, you will see some similarities with Ramadan and Lent. During Ramadan, most people don't eat during the day, and instead eat all their meals at night. This is very similar to a 16/8 fast or even a 20/4 fast, where eating takes place in a small eight or four hour window at night. Depending on the style of Lent a person follows, you may only have one large meal in the day instead of many meals. Or you may only eat for some portion of the week and fast completely on other days. This can also be quite like intermittent fasting schedules. The difference between religious fasts and intermittent fasting are, of course, the purpose but also the timing. Religious fasts often take place for a short period of time like 20-40 days, but intermittent fasting can be a whole lifestyle change, and result in you fasting for years! It's not necessary to do it for the long term, but many people continue it even when they meet their goals for fasting.

There are so many different varieties of intermittent fasting that you'll have and easy way of finding one that fits into your lifestyle. In general, there are the methods that require you to eat in a small window everyday. These are the methods like the 12/12, 14/10, 16/8, and 20/4. In these methods, the first number is how many hours you fast, and the second number is how many hours are in your eating window. You would eat all your meals during that window of time, and during the fasting point, you would just drink liquids. The other types of fasts are those that include 24 hours of fasting between eating days. Some of these do calorie restricted meals during the fasting period so that hunger doesn't become overwhelming. Methods that do the longer 24 hour fast (with or without small meals on fasting days) include alternate day fasts, the 5:2 fast, and a general 24 hour fast. Alternate day fasts and 5:2 fasts can be similar as they take place during the course of one week. However, alternate day fasts require fasting three or four days of the week, alternating your eating days and your fasting days. While the 5:2 fast is eating normally for five days with two days of fasting spread out within the week. The 24 hour fast is one you might do once a week or even just once a month! Whichever fast you choose to do, you'll want to choose one that fits your daily life. We'll discuss these kinds of fasts later in the book.

It's important to mention that intermittent fasting isn't a diet. While people use it to receive health benefits (like they do for dieting), intermittent fasting isn't a diet at all. Most diets are focused on what you eat, however, intermittent fasting is all about when you eat. It focuses on the timing of eating to change your body's current state and bring it more into homeostasis. This can sound a little fantasy-like. Afterall, how can changing the times you eat help? Well, there's a lot of research out there about intermittent fasting, and depending on the type of fasting you follow, intermittent fasting can change your metabolism, insulin levels, and more. Let's explore more about why intermittent fasting works.

I can tell you that you'll lose weight on intermittent fasting and you'll become healthier. But none of that explains why? Why does fasting have such positive reviews and a following? Intermittent fasting works for so many reasons, but the main ones are the fact that it can fit in your daily life, changes some of your physiology, and can result in some caloric restriction.

Diets can cause a lot of changes your life. They often require specific foods that must be eaten. This can be frustrating if you live in an area where some foods aren't available. It can also be frustrating cost wise, as a lot of diet foods can be quite expensive. All of these can impact your motivation to continue dieting. Intermittent fasting doesn't cause this change to your life. You don't have to eat specific types of food when fasting. Nor do you have to spend a fortune following the schedule. All it requires of you is to eat at a specific time of day, and eat healthy meals during your eating window. This can ease the strain of starting a new fasting schedule. This also means that you won't have to do a huge change to your lifestyle.

Chapter 4:
The Benefits of 16:8 Intermittent Fasting

Intermittent fasting techniques, including the 16:8 method, are most commonly used to assist in weight loss by the general population. The method has been tried by thousands of people and also scientifically proven to be a helpful resource in reducing body fat and improving body composition. Weight loss is often considered the number one reason why people opt for a diet and program that utilizes intermittent fasting, in fact.

While a reduction in body fat is definitely one of the best advantages to be mentioned in terms of intermittent fasting, there are more advantages that people gain when they decide that they are going to follow this type of program – especially if they truly commit to it and can implement self-control that ensures they do not give in to cravings.

Body composition refers to a series of features – this includes your body fat percentage and lean muscle mass primarily. A program that utilizes intermittent fasting, along with an appropriate diet plan, will bring down your body fat percentage, and push up your lean muscle mass at the same time.

It is also important to note the benefits that are associated with weight loss for people with an excessive amount of fat distributed throughout their body. Since overweight and obesity is linked to so many chronic diseases that can truly make your life dreadful, losing even small amounts of weight can drastically reduce your risk of these diseases. Additionally, if you have already been diagnosed with a disease associated with obesity, reduced body weight may improve the symptoms that you are experiencing and help you get the disease under control.

Take type 2 diabetes, for example. In one study, scientists describe that factors such as proinflammatory markers, cytokines, hormones, glycerol, and nonesterified fatty acids are all increased among those people who are obese. In turn, these factors all have factors that link them to insulin resistance. When insulin resistance develops, it can continue to progress into type 2 diabetes if the affected person does not implement appropriate preventative measures.

When you develop type 2 diabetes, you become predisposed to many additional risks and complications. In fact, type 2 diabetes can cause severe complications that may not only lead to disability but also become life-threatening. This disease can also affect all of the body's most important organs, including the heart, and can damage various tissues, such as nerves, throughout the body.

In addition to assisting in reducing body weight and bringing down the risks associated with obesity, intermittent fasting has many other benefits that are also worth mentioning.

Through intermittent fasting, cellular changes may occur in the body. This can lead to levels of human growth hormones rising by as much as 500%. This leads to a faster rate of fat burning, while also producing an increase in muscle mass.

It has also been found that intermittent fasting can help to remove waste that has built up in cells within the human body and can also assist in the repair process of cells that have been damaged. This means cells in the body become more efficient in performing their specialized functions.

One study also explains how recent findings from scientists suggest that intermittent fasting helps to improve brain health and may play a crucial role in helping medical experts better understand how diseases like Parkinson's disease and Alzheimer's disease can be prevented in the future.

Furthermore, following an intermittent fasting plan can also help to reduce levels of inflammation within the human body, as well as help to fight against oxidative stress. Both of these factors are known to contribute to numerous chronic diseases significantly and can causes certain molecules to become damaged, which can inhibit their functionality within the body.

In one study, scientists tested how intermittent fasting would work on the brain health and cardiovascular health among a group of laboratory rats. They found significant improvements in various tests used to determine the well-being of these two crucial hormones of the body. The scientists also associated these improvements among the tested laboratory rats with the reduction in oxidative stress that were observed. Additionally, the scientists also observed an improvement in the cellular stress resistance ratings in these rats. What this means is that an intermittent fasting diet can help to reduce the effect that stress has on the body, and help to fight against the existing oxidative damage, often also referred to as free radical damage, that has already occurred.

It is very flexible

Intermittent fasting can be done at any time. It is not as demanding as some diets that cause a massive disruption with your life unnecessarily. Intermittent fasting has no specific duration that it should be done. They can also be mixed as you feel is suitable for your schedule. There is no point where you are boxed into a regiment that is not easy for you to maintain. Intermittent fasting adjusts to the unpredictability of life.

It can also be done anywhere in any part of the world since it is not a certain thing you have to do, it is just restricting food, thus is much simpler and more practice than many diets. Even if you must stop fasting for some time, it is totally okay. It is possible to start fasting again within minutes.

It has a very strong effect

It is the strongest and fastest way to lower insulin levels and insulin resistance. It has more effect than a strict ketogenic diet. It can help you break through stubborn weight loss plateaus. It has no limit thus; there is no maximum amount of time you can be fasting. You can increase your fasting frequency and length to reduce the time you will take to achieve your goal.

Medications, on the other hand, have limits. If you take more medicine than the maximum dosage, it will become toxic and can even lead to death. Even low carbohydrate or fat diets have limits, once you have zero of each, there is not much more you can do to burn fat. Also, some diets can work with some people and not work with others while fasting is for all.

It is favorable

The health benefits of eating a home-cooked meal are many but the time or desire to cook is not always available. Many things occupy most people currently thus; they cannot find residual time in their day when they are not tired. Fasting saves your time, as you do not always have to cook, shop for groceries or prepare ingredients, as you do not eat a lot. It generally makes life a lot simpler. All it involves is doing nothing, which is the easiest thing to do.

It is cost-effective

Organic food such as grass-fed beef and vegetables tower over-processed food nutrient wise. Unfortunately, these organic foods are quite expensive so buying them every day will only thin out your pockets. They are about ten times more costly than processed foods. Feeding on processed foods is clearly the better option cost-wise. Even though a diet is effective, if it is unaffordable, it will not benefit you. Fast here is a clear winner as it is free. Yes, completely free. You do not need to buy any food at all thus, it saves you money. There is nowhere in fasting that you are required to buy expensive food or supplements, or any medication making it the most cost-effective for everyone.

You can still enjoy your life

There are some diets if you decide to start them; you will have to forfeit some foods forever. You may never get to enjoy chocolate or ice cream again which is good for burning fat but not so much for you as a person. This cutback can seem minor but forever cutting them off, is a very long sentence.

Fasting saves the day as it allows you to indulge yourself in such pleasures. This does not mean that you take junk food every day doing that would be destroying yourself, instead, it means enjoying these foods in moderation. Fasting is very accommodating to different situations; you can indulge yourself on the condition that you can accompany them with abstinence. It is all about getting the most optimal balance between healthy and unhealthy foods. You should also maintain the time you are eating and the time that you are not to get maximum benefit.

It is easy to do

Intermittent fasting does not involve difficult planning it is simple to eat nothing and drink water. This makes it better than many diets as it is easier to follow and more effective.

It helps you control mental processes in your body

Intermittent fasting opens your body. You are used to answering any desire your body wants because you eat three meals a day. Intermittent fasting sets you free from your body controlling you. Your body will try to fight back as first but eventually, the rebellion will subside, as it will have adapted. This will release your mind and make it free to concentrate on thing s of more importance as well as bodily repairs.

It also helps improve your brain health. It increases the production of BDNF, which is a protein that guards brain cells against neurological degenerative disorders. You overall brain health will make you feel good.

It improves your physiology

Intermittent fasting significantly reduces the number of calories you take in a day. It is close to impossible to intake the daily-recommended calorie amount in the feeding period you have during fasting. This leads to bodily changes and the burning of fat. It will also help you to burn fat even if you take the regular number of calories, as it will make your body used to use fat instead of carbohydrates for energy.

It improves your hormone reception and control

Intermittent fasting makes the body have low levels of insulin making it sensitive to slight increases. If you take too much sugar, you will eventually become numb to its effects as your insulin levels will be at a constant high. Your insulin reception is very important as insulin is linked to diseases like diabetes. Developments of insulin resistance will hinder the body from accessing fat deposits making you gain fat.

It can synchronize with any diet

No matter what you eat and what you do not eat, you will still be able to do intermittent fasting. It is not locked to certain foods.

It helps prevent heart disease

Blood sugar regulation and reduction of fat are both things that are accomplished by intermittent fasting which improve heart health. It can also reduce the risk of coronary artery heart disease.

It promotes the secretion of the growth hormone

Intermittent fasting increases the secretion of the growth hormone. It is found more in children than adults are but nevertheless it helps a lot. The growth hormone reduces body fat and increases bone and muscle growth. It does this by breaking down glycogen to release glucose into the bloodstream. This helps in promoting fat burning without any muscle loss. The growth hormone is also increased when you get enough sleep and exercise.

Chapter 5:
Can Intermittent Fasting Be Dangerous

Although most people can follow the intermittent fasting diet with minimal side effects and virtually no lasting side effects, some people might find themselves experiencing some. The most likely dangers that you could experience includes:

You Might Struggle to Maintain Blood Sugar Levels

Although the intermittent fasting diet tends to improve blood sugar levels in most people, this is not always true for everyone. Some people who are eating following the intermittent fasting diet may find that their ability to maintain a healthy blood sugar level is compromised.

The reason for why this happens varies. For some people, not eating frequently enough may encourage this to happen. For others, transitioning too quickly or taking on too intense of a fasting cycle too soon, can shock the body which in turn causes a strange fluctuation in blood sugar levels.

You Might Experience Hormonal Imbalances

A certain degree of fasting, especially when you build up to it, can support you in having healthier hormone levels. However, for some people, intermittent fasting may lead to an unhealthy imbalance of hormones. This can result in a whole slew of different hormone-based symptoms, such as headaches, fatigue, and even menstrual problems in women.

Again, the reason for the hormonal imbalance varies. For some people, particularly those who are already at risk of experiencing hormonal imbalances, intermittent fasting can trigger these imbalances to take place. For others, it could go back to what they are consuming during the eating windows. Eating meals that are not rich in nutrients and vitamins can result in you not having enough nutrition to support your hormonal levels.

If you begin experiencing hormonal imbalances when you eat the intermittent fasting diet, it is essential that you stop and consult your doctor right away. Discovering where the shortcomings are and how you can correct them is vital. Having imbalanced hormones for too long can lead to diseases and illnesses that require constant life-long attention.

Headaches

A decrease in your blood sugar level and the release of stress hormones by your brain as a result of going without food are possible causes of headaches during the fasting window. Problems may also be a clear message from your body telling you that you are very low on water and getting dehydrated. This may happen if you are completely engrossed in your daily activities, and you forget to drink the required amount of water your body needs during fasting.

To handle headaches, ensure you stay well hydrated throughout your fasting window. Keep in mind that exceeding the required amount of water per day may also result in adverse effects. Reducing your stress level can also keep headaches away.

Some people find that the transitioning period includes many headaches. These headaches are often a result of you being hungry as your body adjusts to your new eating schedule. Typically, these headaches are dull and should be manageable. If it is not, you may be experiencing excessively low blood sugars. If your headache is too intense, refrain from fasting and eat. It is better to skip your fasting cycle and eat if you are experiencing negative side effects, than it is to attempt to stick it out and experience adverse or potentially dangerous side effects.

If you are experiencing chronic headaches, you may also be experiencing dehydration. Dehydration is common in most people, but it can be especially prevalent in those who are fasting. Typically, eating encourages us to drink, too. This is how we "wash it down." When you are not eating, you may also forget to drink water. Setting reminders to drink water and remember to get at least 3L a day can support you in overcoming headaches that may be caused by dehydration.

Cravings

During your fasting periods, you might find that you have higher levels of desires than usual. This often happens because you are telling yourself that you cannot have any food, so suddenly you start craving many different foods. This is because all you are thinking about is food. As you think about food, you will begin to think about the different types of food that you like and that you want. Then, the cravings start.

Early on, you may also find yourself craving more sweets or carbs because your body is searching for an energy hit through glucose. While you do not want to have excessive levels of sugar during your eating window, as this is bad for blood sugar, you can always have some. The ability to satisfy your cravings is one of the benefits of eating a diet that is not as restrictive as some other foods are.

From a psychological angle, cravings are intensified because of a feeling of being deprived of what you love to eat. For example, telling you to keep away from eating chocolate will somehow make you want to eat chocolate even more because you are unconsciously trying to overcome the feeling of being deprived. Stopping yourself from eating at the usual times you have conditioned your body to received food will naturally make you crave food more at those typical eating times.

To effectively handle your cravings, keep your mind off of food during the fasting window. Ensure that during your eating window, you indulge a bit with what your body craves. This will help to dampen the longing for that thing. Remember that you are not dieting, but fast, so you shouldn't worry unnecessarily over what you eat. Your focus should be on when you eat.

Low Energy

A feeling of lethargy is not uncommon during fasting, especially at the start. This is your body's natural reaction to switching its source of energy from glucose in your meals to fat stored in your body. So, expect to feel a little less energized in your first few weeks of starting with intermittent fasting.

To troubleshoot the feeling of lethargy, try as much as possible to stay away from overly strenuous activities. Keep things low key. Spending more time sleeping or just relaxing is another right way to ensure that your energy reserves are not depleted too quickly. The first few weeks are not the time to test your limits or push yourself.

Foul Mood

You may find yourself being on edge during fasting, even if you are someone who is naturally predisposed to being good-natured. The reason for the feeling of edginess is straightforward. You are hungry, yet you won't eat, and you are struggling to keep your cravings in check, plus, you may already be feeling tired and sluggish. Add all of these to the internal hormone changes due to the sharp decline in your blood sugar levels, and it's no wonder why you may be in such a foul mood. Tempers can easily flare up, and you may be quick to become irritated. This is normal when beginning a fasting lifestyle.

To effectively troubleshoot this, do all you can to keep away from irritable people and situations. If you consider someone annoying, do your best to stay out of their company or else they are more than likely to set you on edge. Find a way to deliberately focus your attention on things that easily trigger a feeling of happiness in you. Consciously seeking ways to be appreciative of the things around you, as well as to being grateful about the simple things of life, will go a long way toward keeping you from being easily irritated.

To handle this cold feeling, you can put on extra warm clothing, stay in friendly places, or drink a hot cup of unsweetened coffee. Taking a hot shower can also reduce the coldness.

Excess Urination

Fasting tends to make you visit the bathroom more frequently than usual. This is an expected side effect since you are drinking more water and other liquids than before. Avoiding water to reduce the number of times you use the bathroom is not a good idea at all, no matter how you look at it. Cutting down water intake while you are fasting will make your body become dehydrated very quickly. If that happens, losing weight will be the least of your problems. Whatever you do, do not avoid drinking water when you are fasting. Doing that is paving the way for a humongous health disaster waiting to happen. You don't want to do that.

The best way to handle excess urination is to stay close to a bathroom or a toilet wherever you find yourself throughout the day. You should urinate when the need arises. There is no other healthy shortcut to it.

People who are intermittently fasting tend to drink a lot of water in between eating windows. That is if they remember to. Often, water is used as a way to fill up your stomach to avoid feeling hungry throughout the day. It can also support you in overcoming heartburn. As a result, water is a popular option for people who are intermittently fasting.

At first, you may even find yourself going as often as twice an hour! There truly is no way around this, as water is essential and you do not want to decrease your intake. This will likely be a symptom that you experience on an ongoing basis, but you should see it as a good sign. This proves that you are well-hydrated and taking good care of your body.

Heartburn, Bloating, and Constipation

Your stomach is responsible for producing stomach acid, which is used to break down food and trigger the digestion process. When you eat frequent meals, unusually large meals, regularly, your body is used to producing high amounts of stomach acid to break down your food. As you transition to a fasting diet, your stomach has to get used to not producing as much stomach acid.

You might also notice an increase in constipation and bloating. People who eat regularly consume high amounts of fiber and proteins that support a healthy digestion process. When you switch to the intermittent fasting cycle, you can still eat a high volume of fiber and protein. However, early on, you might find that you forget to. As you discover the right eating habits that work for you, it may take some time for you to get used to finding ways to work in enough fiber and protein to keep your digestion flowing.

Heartburn may not be a widespread adverse effect, but it does sometimes occur in some individuals. Your stomach produces highly concentrated acids to help break down the foods you consume. But when you are fasting, there is no food in your stomach to be broken down, even though acids have already been produced for that purpose. This may lead to heartburn.

Bloating and constipation usually go hand in hand and can be very discomforting to individuals who suffer from it due to fasting.

Heeding the advice to drink adequate amounts of water usually keeps bloating and constipation in check. Heartburn typically resolves itself quickly, but you can take an antacid tablet or two if it persists. You may also consider eating fewer spicy foods when you break your fast.

You Might Experience Low Energy and Irritability

Until now, your body has been used to having a constant stream of energy pouring in all day long. From the time you wake up until the time you go to bed, it has been receiving some form of power from the foods that you eat. So, when you stop eating regularly, your body grows confused. It has to learn to create its energy rather than rely on the heat being offered to it by the food that you are eating.

Depending on how you are eating, your body may also be growing used to consuming fat as a fuel source rather than carbohydrates. This means that, in addition to losing its primary energy source, it also has to switch how it consumes energy and where it comes from. This can lead to lowered energy for a while. Do things that exert the least amount of energy. If you are someone who regularly exercises and works out, reducing the amount that you work out or switching to a more relaxed workout like yoga can help you during the transition period.

You Might Start Feeling Cold

As you begin to adjust to your intermittent fasting diet, you might find that your fingers and toes get quite cold. This happens because blood flow towards your fat stores is increasing, so blood flow to your extremities reduces slightly. This supports your body in moving fat to your muscles so that it can be burned as a fuel to keep your energy levels up.

Lowered blood sugars from fasting can also lead to cold extremities. More so, it makes them feel more sensitive to the cold. Staying warm with tea, hot showers, and extra layers can help overcome this coldness. If you notice that it is particularly prominent or that it spreads beyond your fingers and toes, you might want to adjust your diet to ensure that you are not experiencing chronic low blood sugars. This will ensure that you continue effectively managing your symptoms without experiencing adverse or dangerous side effects from intermittent fasting.

You Might Find Yourself Overeating

The chances for overeating during the break of the fast are high, especially for beginners. Understandably, you will feel starving after going without food for longer than you are used to. It is this hunger that causes some people to eat hurriedly and surpass their standard meal size and average caloric intake. For others, overeating may be as a result of uncontrollable appetite. Hunger may push some people to prepare too much food for breaking their fast, and if they don't have a grip on their desire, they will continue to eat even when they are satiated. Overeating or binging when you break your fast will make it difficult to reach your goal of optimal health and fitness.

An excellent way to tackle this is by making adequate plans ahead of time and sticking to those plans. Plan the quantity of food to be prepared well ahead of the eating window. Take into consideration the type of food as well as the meal size to be eaten. Although it may not be feasible to continually eat only fatty foods, increasing the frequency as well as the number of healthy fats in your diet will help you to feel satiated quickly.

During the windows where you can eat, you might find yourself eating as much as you possibly can. This is often a natural response to the feelings of hunger that you have experienced during your fasting cycle.

Choosing healthier options and eating mindfully is a good way to overcome overeating habits. This can support you in selecting options that are going to nourish and help your body, as well as prevent overeating. When you eat slowly and mindfully, you can recognize when you are no longer hungry. As a result, you can set down the fork and stop eating. Eating healthier options and eating slowly are the best ways to avoid overeating so that you do not waste your fasting benefits on an excessively unhealthy diet during your eating windows.

Hunger Pangs

People who start intermittent fasting may initially feel quite hungry. This is especially common if you are the type of person who tends to eat regular meals daily.

If you start feeling hungry, you can choose to wait it out if you have an eating window right around the corner. However, if there is a more extended waiting period or you are feeling excessively hungry, you should eat. Feeling hungry to the point that it becomes uncomfortable or distracting is not helpful and will not support you in successfully taking on the intermittent fasting diet. This is a pronounced side effect of going without food for longer than you are accustomed to.

For many people, their bodies have been conditioned to eat at certain regular intervals. So, at those intervals, their hunger hormones kick into action and stimulate a feeling of hunger. They either respond by eating a full meal or grabbing a quick snack. It is almost impossible not to feel very hungry when you attempt to break this pattern. Introducing fasting into your lifestyle is going to make you hungry. There are no two ways about it, and I'm not going to lie to you. The intensity of hunger is even higher when you are just starting. Hunger tests your resolve and mental toughness, especially in your first few days. This is the point where many will give up and walk away from their dreams and aspirations. But if you stay true to your resolve, hunger has a way of waning over time.

Chapter 6:
How to stay motivated when practicing intermittent fasting

To achieve your weight loss and fitness goals, it is quintessential that you stick to the diet for at least a month to see any positive changes. If you want to stick to this diet, then you need to be self-motivated. There will be days when you don't have the motivation to keep going. In this section, you'll learn about specific simple tips that will come in handy whenever you are running low on motivation.

Set Your Goals

Before you decide to start a diet, it is time to analyze why you want to start a diet. What are the reasons why you wish to diet? What are your goals? You might want to lose weight, improve your fitness levels, or even lead a healthier life. Reasons tend to vary from one individual to another. If you don't set any goals for yourself, you will quickly lose motivation after a couple of weeks of dieting. However, while setting goals. There are a couple of simple things you must keep in mind. Ensure that the goals you set are specific, measurable, attainable, relevant, and time bound. Even if one of these ingredients is missing, then the chances of attaining such a goal will reduce.

If you set any unrealistic goals for yourself, you are setting yourself up for failure. For instance, a goal like, "I want to lose 40 pounds within four weeks," is quite unrealistic. By setting such lofty goals, you are setting yourself up for failure. When you cannot attain such an impossible goal, you will be demotivated, and you will quickly lose interest in dieting altogether. Any goal that you set needs to have a time limit. If you don't set a time limit for yourself, procrastination can creep in, and the likelihood of sticking to the diet will also reduce. Therefore, an ideal goal would be, "I want to lose two to three pounds every month."

Pick a date

You must always pick a date to start this diet. Don't be in a hurry and think that you can get started with this diet right away. There are a couple of things you need to do before you can begin to diet. For instance, you will need to stock up on all the ingredients you require to cook keto-friendly meals. Apart from this, you will also need to prepare yourself mentally to get started with the new diet. All this takes planning and preparation. You cannot skip these two necessary steps if you want to stick to the diet in the long run. When you opt for a specific date, ensure that you start dieting, from that day itself. Don't procrastinate, and don't tell yourself that you can start dieting from tomorrow. That "tomorrow" might never have come around. Maybe you can mark the date on your calendar to remind yourself that you are supposed to start with your diet.

Meal Plan

To ensure that you stick to the diet, you will need a meal plan. The good news is you don't have to create a meal plan for yourself. There is a detailed meal plan in this book. You can use it to get started with your new diet. Ensure that you include plenty of variety. Whenever you plan, the meals out for a week. If the food you eat starts getting repetitive, you will quickly lose interest to stick to your diet. Also, when you have a meal plan in place, it becomes easier to shop for groceries. If you know that you have a healthy meal waiting for you at home, the temptation of eating out will also reduce.

Make Calories Count

A common reason why a lot of people lose interest in dieting is because of hunger pangs. Ensure that you make every calorie count. Don't binge on unhealthy foods and instead, opt for nutrient-dense options. When your tummy is full, the urge to snack on junk food will reduce. If your daily calorie intake is 1800 calories, then ensure that you manage to eat at least two well-balanced, hearty meals. You can undoubtedly blow this calorie count by binging on a pint of ice cream, but it will do you no good.

Grocery Shopping

It is time to clean your pantry! Raid your kitchen and discard any unhealthy foods you find. Get rid of all cookies, cakes, chocolates, sodas, and other foods you must not eat while on the keto diet. Out of sight and out of mind is the best policy when it comes to dieting. If temptations surround you, the urge to give in will increase. Instead, stock up your pantry will keto-friendly ingredients. Once you have all the ingredients you need, it becomes easier to cook as well. Always prepare a grocery list before you go shopping and stick to this list.

Visualization

Whenever you are running low on motivation, remind yourself of the reasons why you started dieting. Think about the goals you want to attain. Start visualizing your goals. Think about how wonderful and happy you will feel when you attain your goals. While doing this, also think about how disappointed you would be if you didn't attain those same goals. While visualizing your goals, try to make the visualization as detailed as you possibly can. If you want, you can create a visualization board for yourself. Take a sheet of paper, make a note of your goal on it, and place it somewhere visible. Glance at it daily. It will act as a subconscious reminder for your mind. Fill this board up with positive affirmations, quotes, or even images that motivate you to stick to the diet.

A Dieting Buddy

The best way to ensure that you stay on track and stick to your diet is to find a dieting partner for yourself. Maybe you can start this diet with your partner, a friend, a loved one, family member, or anyone else. If you want, there are plenty of online forums; you can join and interact with others who are going through the same situation that you are in. When you do this, you will realize that you aren't alone. This, by itself, will give you plenty of motivation to keep going.

By following the simple tips given in this section, you can ensure that your motivation levels stay high as you get started with this diet.

Chapter 7:
Why our modern diet is wrong

We all know we need to eat healthily. We also know that we need to limit how much soda, drinks, processed foods, sugar we eat. But even though we know these things, it doesn't mean they are easy to follow.

According to a recent Food and Health Survey conducted by Psychology Today, 52 percent of Americans believe it is easier to calculate their taxes than know how to eat healthily. Too many people are having problems with this modern tax code, which means that many people have trouble figuring out how to eat the right foods for them.

We live in a country that is battling obesity. More than one-third of people in the United States are considered obese, and many are also considered to be overweight. However, these statistics do not show the full picture. Three out of three adults are considered overweight or obese, meaning that most people will fall into this category.

Why are these statistics so bad? Many factors contribute to obesity. One major culprit is classic American food. There has been a significant decline in the quality of our food as we have gone from a nation dependent on food from local farms to a nation that produces most of the food. This transition has increased our appetite for food because it is available now.

Also, many readily available and easily consumed foods are high in fat, sugar, and calories. All of these things help increase weight. From the sugary snacks, we get from the restroom to all the food chains around us, the quality of the food, and the amount we eat have dramatically changed. We can eat healthy foods without stopping if we want to, which is why obesity is so prevalent in our culture.

The first thing to look at is the amount of food we eat. The number of calories everyone needs may vary from person to person. Ingredients include your genes, your level of activity, your overall health, height, age, and gender. However, the target number used in food labels is about 2000 calories per day. This number is already fairly high for those living a stable life. It is also possible to eat 2000 calories or more in one sitting if you go out to eat.

Although the food out quickly us pushing the number of calories, it is also possible to eat too much when I eat at home. It is important to learn how to start eating what we need to work on, rather than eating because something tastes good, or we get bored, or tired.

To calculate the average daily calories consumed by Americans, organizations are examining the amount of food available per capita that shows the amount of food consumed. In the United States, this ends up around 3800 calories per day. Even when you take into account the fact that some of these foods are lost or discarded daily rather than eaten, the average American consumes 2700 calories per day. This is the approach that everyone will need, even if they lead an active lifestyle and not many Americans.

Now, we need to also discuss the quality of food most Americans eat. Growing up, most of us learn from our parents and teachers about what is good and what is not. Fruits and vegetables are seen as such well, and sugar and sweets are bad. The rest of the diet may not be as good as before, but they were good in moderation. Although we have been taught about healthy eating at an early age, it is still culturally difficult to follow these tips.

According to the Agricultural Department in the U.S., the top six sources of calories for most Americans are fruit-based sweets, yeast, poultry, sports/energy drinks, and alcoholic beverages. Remember that healthy fruits and vegetables are not listed. In the top five lists, the most common foods Americans eat are refined fruits and sugar. It is estimated that only 8% of the average American diet consists of fruits and vegetables.

According to a study by the US Department of Agriculture (USDA) in 2010, nuts, meat, and eggs make up 21% of these foods; oils and fats make up 23%, and calorie sweeteners make up 15%. Food that is not good for us constitutes 61 percent of our diet.

The time of day we eat is also important. Most Americans live a busy lifestyle and do not have time to sit and eat a balanced diet. In effect, they eat walking, usually in some areas unhealthy, or eat at night when their metabolism is slow. Besides, many Americans are sitting in bed and eating unhealthy snacks while watching television. Sometimes the diet is high, so we eat non-stop food.

It is important to learn the steps necessary to limit the amount of food we take each day. It is tempting to eat readily available foods. But, if you want to get back to your health and get better in a good way, it is important to stay away from classic American food and choose something good for you.

When you hear fasting, you can think of people who go for weeks without eating for religious reasons. You may think it is unhealthy or incapable of doing it because you love food. But intermittent fasting is different from religious fasting, although they share common ideas.

Indirect fasting is limiting your calorie intake in parts of the day or not eating too much on certain days. Your body still gets the nutrients it needs, but you eat fewer calories, so keeping it simple gravity. Some of the various types of fast cot will have discussed later in this book.

The reason this diet is successful is that it is effective in reducing the amount of fat in your body, as well as the number of calories you eat. Since you are reducing the time allowed to eat or reduce your calorie intake during certain days of the week, it is easy to lower your total calorie count. You can also choose how much time you would like to do quickly. Some people choose to do it for a month or more while others may fit their lifestyle, so they stick to it in the long run.

Avoid Unhealthy Eating Habits

After dinner, you are overweight, but you can't resist ordering desserts. If your stomach is hungry all day, then sweeten yourself until you fall asleep. Or maybe you can always eat something, such as walking, parking, or driving.

If any of these situations seem common, you can use your eating habits in preparation. They can all show unhealthy habits and can lose weight successfully for a long time.

Listen to Your Body

Anyone struggling with food allergies will develop a disruptive behavior that nutritionists can call. Poor eating habits can take many forms, from eating poorly to developing obesity and eating disorders, bulimia, or anorexia.

To allow yourself to want to lose weight and develop a healthy diet, your first step should be to accept your body and be proud that you are a member of a Weight Loss Program to keep your body healthy.

One of the best ways to regulate your eating habits is to stay active - learn how to eat when you are hungry and stop smoking after eating. It is easy to say, but with a little education, you will learn how to control your calories but not feel lost.

No One Is Perfect

Your goal should be to remain neutral, not perfect. Do not have physical cravings for food that can lead to physical inactivity, which can lead to many stomach ailments and eating disorders.

This book will help you improve your diet and create a diet plan that includes your favorite foods, including low-fat or healthy foods, to keep you healthy and satisfied. You need to slowly change your diet and improve your lifestyle to get the best results.

One powerful example to avoid eating is to put away a lot of calories from your face. Resistance is impossible when the food is under your nose!

But don't give up. You do not have to resist the urge to enter. What to do is to prevent parties and places with lots of junk food. Before you begin your first meal, please do a "stomach test": are you hungry, or do you just crave for something to eat?

If the food is like putting some oil in a container, our lives will be easier, but eating is more than an empty container.

Many cultural, behavioral, emotional, social, and environmental factors can help us determine how much time we spend in the stress of the job, and such hard experiences can make us start eating.

Consider whether you decide to eat or not, rather than decide without being conscious or unconscious. Can you choose what to eat? It will be easier if you start choosing a healthy diet - you will have to regain the spirit as you experience the benefits of your tradition.

How to Change Bad Habits

Change is not always easy, especially for long-term behavior. So here are some tips to help you put away these bad habits into practice:

Develop a plan to manage your daily contact with them. Decide how to address your weaknesses to be aware of the situation.

Replace unhealthy foods with good food. If eating at night is your weakness, please give yourself a small snack in the evening.

Too much sleep - it can slow down your eating time!

Reduce TV viewing. You don't have time to try meals, and you have time to exercise.

Set goals that are realistic for you. Not sure what will happen to you. Slowly change your habit of taking drugs.

Thinking positive, negative thoughts like "I can't" or "I'm tired and distracted" can enable you to succeed in your course. Write inspirational ideas and read them when you need help to focus on your goals.

Find your friends or hire supportive friends to maximize your chances of success. Studies have shown that support is essential to the success of behavioral changes and barriers.

Chapter 8:
16:8 Diet and Do's and Don'ts

Adjust Your Diet Plan as You Go

I will share an excellent diet plan with you in this book, and it is perfectly normal and okay to follow the plan for the full two weeks that I have designed it for. Even after that, you may continue with the program in order to experience more benefits, such as reduced body weight and to gain an improvement in your overall health.

Now, at the same time, I do want to note that following one single plan over an extended period of time will often not offer you the best results that you could achieve through intermittent fasting.

The thing is every person is different – you are unique. For this reason, a specific meal plan that works for you will likely not be ideal for every other person.

This means that the diet program proposed in this book might be able to work, but you may need to make some modifications as you go along in order to achieve the specific goals that you have in mind with the program that you are implementing.

Sure, you are not a dietician with years of experience in the industry, which really does make it somewhat harder for you to develop an appropriate diet plan that will suit you and help you achieve the goals you are striving toward. This, however, does not necessarily mean that it will be impossible for you to make simple adjustments in order to reach those weight loss goals.

Here's an example: you follow the diet plan that I have provided you here to the point, and prepare the specific meals that I have provided you with. Even though you implement these meal plans every day and you avoid binge eating, you will find that you are not losing a lot of weight. In this case, there might not be an appropriate caloric deficit in your weight management plan.

Don't Overlook The Importance Of Exercise In a Weight Loss Strategy

I have seen a lot of people start with an intermittent fasting plan and end up complaining that the program is not working for them. The same person would then tell me that they do not have a very physical lifestyle.

You must have read the topic where I explained how intermittent fasting is used for weight loss already by now, so you should understand that without expending calories each day, you won't be able to lose that excess fat that has accumulated inside your body.

Expending calories mean being physically active. Unfortunately, quite a large percentage of the worldwide population are living sedentary lifestyles. With a sedentary lifestyle, you are really "paving the way" for weight gain. If you are not physically active, you won't be able to burn an adequate number of calories each day for weight loss to be possible in the first place.

The more you exercise, the more calories you will burn, of course. At the same time, you should be sure not to overdo things in terms of physical activity. There really is no use in causing yourself injury due to over-training – this will only lead to temporary disability and will make training harder for the next few days (sometimes weeks or months if you suffer a more serious injury).

It is best to create a balanced exercise plan for yourself and then test it out. Listen to your body and understand when you are pushing yourself, as well as when you have some extra capacity available to up your game at the gym.

You will have to take your daily calorie consumption into account here – we did discuss how you can calculate your ideal daily calorie requirement in a previous section. This data will definitely come in handy here. Calculate an appropriate exercise plan that will ensure your daily caloric expenditure is reached through physical exercise just in case you exceed your daily caloric intake.

Deal with Hunger Pangs Like a Boss

Let's tackle a topic that you will likely face yourself. Hunger pangs are something that we all experience when we first start out with an intermittent fasting plan. You suddenly have to get your body adjusted to an entirely new way of eating. No longer do you get up in the morning and cook up some eggs and bacon. You have to get up and drink water, or perhaps have a cup of coffee, but you'll have to wait until the afternoon before you get to have your first meal.

So, the question now is, should you give in to the temptations that you will be experiencing, especially during those first few days, or should you implement an appropriate strategy to help you better cope with these hunger pangs and the cravings that you are going to experience.

There are different strategies that you can use to cope with your cravings. One would be to drink a glass of water if you feel hungry and you can feel those cravings building up. This is an effective strategy for lots of people, but not for everyone, of course. If you find that plain water or even filtered water does not work well for you, then I suggest you try some fizzy water (carbonated water). Be sure not to opt for carbonated water with added sweetening agents, as these are loaded with some carbs. Rather just opt for plain sparkling water. The carbonation in the water can help to make you feel full for a while to ensure you can get through to your eating window without giving in to your temptations.

It is important that you are patient and practice self-control when cravings start building up. Giving in to these cravings should not be considered okay now-and-then, as this will break the fasting window and it will yield less effective results compared to ensuring you last until you are inside of your eating window.

Avoid Eating These Foods

With intermittent fasting, a lot of people tend to follow their usual eating habits in terms of the specific foods that they put on their plate during each meal, expecting that they will lose weight just because they have fasted during the morning, night, and a part of the afternoon.

While intermittent fasting may help to improve metabolism and support digestive function that will ultimately improve your ability to lose weight, the food you eat still counts. As you might have noted, the meal plans that I shared with you in this cookbook generally combines a range of healthy foods in order to ensure you get the nutrients you need without loading up on too many carbs. I did include a lot of delicious options that you can try out.

Just as there are a lot of foods that you can surely include in your diet to help you lose that extra weight that is causing you concern, there are also some foods that you should always try to avoid if your goal is to lose weight.

Below, I would like to share some of the most important foods that you should try to exclude from your diet in order to improve the results you are able to achieve when you implement the recipes and meal plans I have provided you within this book.

· Fried foods, of course, should be at the top of my list. There is no doubt that fried foods are one particularly common reason for the world to be so obese. Millions of people eat fried foods as much as every day. This does not only cause them to gain in weight, but also to experience a rise in cholesterol levels, be at a higher risk of heart disease, and more.

· Fast foods, along with fried foods, since most chains that offer fast foods tend to deep fry their food in the worst types of oil and fat to make them more 'tasty' for the general public. Unfortunately, this also adds more fat to your belly, thighs, arms, and other areas of your body.

· Corn is another food that really isn't the best choice for people who are trying to lose weight. Sure, it is not an unhealthy food, but consider the fact that this is a type of grain that is relatively high in sugar. The sugar spike experienced when you eat corn leads to the release of insulin, triggering inflammation and taking you one step closer to the dreadful complications of insulin resistance.

In addition to all of these, be sure to be wary of added sugars in everything you eat. For example, if you visit your local supermarket and grab a healthy bar to use as the food to break your fast, the fact that the word "healthy" appears on the bar does not necessarily mean it is truly healthy.

Always look at the ingredients of what you buy and what you will be putting into your body. Making your own healthy energy bars at home might be a better solution as well.

Chapter 9:
Potential downsides and who should not fast

Setbacks

Setbacks are sometimes inevitable when it comes to any type of life change, intermittent fasting is no different. Setbacks can include general fasting knowledge, lack of discipline, willpower, self-control, fear of missing out, lack of planning or procrastination, illnesses, that may or may not include medications, that prevent this type of fasting, lack of motivation, resistance to change, YOU, and much more.

Practice Makes Perfect
Getting acquainted with the process of fasting in general and testing your chosen time frames for your feeding and fasting windows can be a difficult time if you are used to eating many meals/snacks daily. Being motivated to continue to develop in this change is just as important as anything else that comes along with this change. Live each day uniquely, such that, if something does not work out well one day, you may change your process the next day until you have feeding and fasting windows that work well with your daily routine schedule. Mind over matter, you matter, so make sure your mind continues to know this fact to ensure you aren't resistant to this change.

Don't be Weak
During the initial change stage, there must be an increased amount of willpower, discipline, and self-control. You will be required to practice your self-control around others who are NOT on an intermittent fasting lifestyle. A person needs to have the willpower to refrain from ingesting calories during their fasting window. You need to have the discipline to create these time frames and stick to them, and when the feeding and/or

fasting windows are broken, create consequences for yourself to ensure it does not happen again until it does not happen anymore.

Fear of Missing Out (FOMO)
Because of how you are used to living your life, sometimes you may feel like you are missing out on the fun surrounding social and/or family eating events, but consider the fact that you are making this change to perfect how you feel and how you look to ensure you are around for a long life to enjoy life. Family and friends may not be on this lifestyle and either may or may not support this change. Alcohol should be consumed in moderation. If you choose to drink alcohol, two or less daily drinks should be the max. Choose non-sugary spirits and alcohol volume dry wines to ensure you are getting the best buzz for your choice.

Holidays will more than likely be the biggest change for you and the biggest day to test you when new to this lifestyle. Holidays are all about eating and tasting everything with family and friends and making memories. Try to prepare in advance by either assisting with cooking to ensure meals are ready before/during your feeding window and choose your favorites to ensure you are satisfied and not as vulnerable after your feeding window closes. The holidays will test you.

Prepare, Don't Procrastinate
Preparation is key. Now that you have decided on your feeding window, ALWAYS, make sure you have your meals/snacks readily available during these times. Stay ahead of your schedule by a day or more, ensure you pack your meals/snacks even if you will be away from home so that you can effectively maintain this healthy lifestyle. Even if you plan to be home, always make sure you take at least a few snack options with your wherever you go. By planning and preparing in this manner, you are sure not to ever go on without anything to eat. It is better for you to maximize your feeding window.

Not Reading Labels and Controlling Portions
Although your calories are NOT restricted when intermittent fasting, eating too much of even healthy foods can lead to weight gain no matter

the type of diet/lifestyle you are following. To prevent this type of setback meal plan, use portion control, be consistent with choosing the most nutritious food choices, and measure your foods to ensure you are not eating too many servings in one meal.

Nonsense from Others

There are times in life when it's better to keep your goals to yourself. Keep your goals away from negative people, specifically keep negative people away from your goals and out of your life. To be successful in many things in life, you need a support system, which does not include negative people. You need someone who can cheer you on, someone who can motivate you, someone, who may be willing to join you, someone who doesn't add to your problems by persuading you to do what is against your goals. If you have negative-thinking people around you, do not tell them your plan of intermittent fasting.

Myths vs. Facts

Understanding the differences is important to your success. Myths may create too much negative space and create room for failure. Facts should educate you enough to keep you motivated and interested in proving that you can be successful with intermittent fasting. It is a myth that not eating 5-6 meals a day will ruin your metabolism and muscle mass. It is a myth that intermittent fasting causes muscle loss, encourages overeating, causes food cravings, causes nutrient deficiencies, and is unnatural and unhealthy for your body. It is a fact that intermittent fasting creates consistencies in eating habits, helps with fat loss, weight management, and promotes a healthy system. Myths are generally kept alive for financial interest.

The Dreaded Scale

Weighing yourself daily is normal for some people, especially those who have tried so many diets, fads, supplements, diet drinks, food restrictions, etc. so this won't be any different. It is normal to want to weigh yourself daily, but this is not healthy for the success of living an intermittent fasting lifestyle. Weigh yourself one day out of the week, same day, same time, same platform and place of scale, same clothes or no clothes, etc. Weighing yourself should be part of your routine. Choose a day and time and stick to it, BUT don't get too caught up on numbers.

Intermittent fasting burns fat as fuel so the scale may not move as fast as you would expect, but to counterbalance this, you will be losing continues measurements, so be sure to take your measurements and pictures of yourself from all angles. Don't let the numbers on the scale be the thing that makes you quit intermittent fasting, observe the fitting of your clothes, keep note of your measurements and look at how your numbers drop, and create grids of before and after pictures to compare your weight success.

Social Media

It's very easy to get caught up on what you see and read on social media. The many transformation stories are fabulous and sound too simple, easy, and those before and after pictures, are like heaven to your eyes. You see that one person that you are following whose before picture looks just like you currently, and you wonder. Why haven't I gotten there? Why did it only take her 3 months to look like this? What am I doing wrong? Am I doing anything right? Is my process working? Is intermittent fasting having any positive effects on me?

Illnesses

Lastly, illness could be considered a potential temporary setback, or even sometimes permanent. If this occurs, please see your medical professional on advice on how to move forward with this change or not, depending on what is recommended, sometimes it may just be a change in the times or of something similar.

The Lifestyle Change and Daily Routine

Creating Habits

There is a huge adaptive component needed to be successful in changing your lifestyle to include intermittent fasting. The most important aspect is learning to create a habit, being consistent regardless of what life has to offer for you. Habits are hard to create. To create a habit, write down your daily routine and stick with it. Share your daily routine with family members to ensure they know what your new routine consists of and what it does not include. Commit to at least 21 days initial to make the habits and routine stick and make it as simple as possible.

Your response to things is what creates habits. With intermittent fasting, it is critical that during your fasting windows, if you get hungry or have cravings, that you gravitate to water, coffee, and tea, this response will become an effective response to hunger, which will create a successful habit to maintain intermittent fasting.

Skipping Days

As you begin to attempt to create habits, skipping days meant for intermittent fasting will not prove to be effective. Once you start this change, it is critical that regardless of weekends, holidays, social events, and more, that you make this routine so that your habits begin to stick. Skipping days restarts the process for your body and mind, and restarting intermittent fasting every time is NOT a habit that you should adopt. You must be consistent. There is no benefit in putting your mind and/or body through this repeatedly without committing to making it a habit.

Make it Simple

To make this a simple change, decide on your feeding and fasting windows as close to your life schedule now. Create a few meals and snack options and stick to a limited list, to begin with for meal planning and shopping; don't have too many options. Too many options could make this change seem impossible when it doesn't have to be, so keep everything simple. You don't have to journal every day if you don't just automatically gravitate to it. You don't have to measure foods and meal preps all the time, do what you can when you can, don't put too much pressure on anything.

Disruption in the social part of eating

Eating from time immemorial has been a highly social activity. Special occasions, celebrations, milestone completion and other major occasions all involve sharing food with people close to you. Intermittent fasting can interfere with your social hangouts as you are eating pattern changes and may not match the regular one. Due to the short window, you must eat you maybe the odd one out in events where everyone is busy eating and drinking merrily. You will miss out on many events that involve eating such as lunch meetings, family suppers, and romantic dinners late at night among many others

Being low on energy

Though the hunger goes away after some time, life is still unpredictable. You may find yourself engaging in an activity that will make you hungrier and eventually unproductive until the hunger passes. You may be already used to eating a lot of snacks in a day and stop abruptly because of fasting; this can lead to some side effects. Those side effects include headaches, bad temper, and lack of energy, headaches, constipation, and poor concentration. It can also reduce your motivation to be active.

Overeating

The restriction of food for a certain time in intermittent fasting is a very good practice. However, people take advantage of the eating window and eat a lot. They end up taking in more calories than they require thus undoing the calorie deficit created by the fasting period. It is very tempting to do this but is highly advised against.

It can lead to some digesting complications

Taking a large meal very fast causes digestion problem. In the eating window in intermittent fasting, people tend to have larger meals translating to longer digesting time required. This leads to increased stress to your digestive tract resulting in indigestion and bloating. This has a bigger effect on people with sensitive guts.

It is not suited for everyone

This type of fasting can cause a negative impact on your health if you have a medical condition. For example, people who are hypoglycemic require glucose throughout the day thus intermittent fasting cannot benefit them.

It may have some long-term negative health outcomes

If the fasting regimen is done, in a way, that largely restricts protein and energy there is a high chance that it may cause issues with fertility in women, cause electrolyte abnormalities and create nutrient deficiencies. Intermittent fasting is associated with menstruation, early menopause, and fertility issues. Research shows that on top of reducing body size it can reduce ovary size thus affecting reproduction.

There is potential weight gain

Intermittent fasting reduces the body's dependence on carbohydrates for energy and makes it rely more on fats. This increases the breakdown of stored fats. The body can develop physiological adaptations as a response to the extreme reduction of energy intake in the body. In simple terms, it means that you may not be able to maintain your new weight or gain even more weight after severe food restriction.

It can cause the refeeding syndrome

This is a dangerous and deadly condition that can occur if your malnutrition. It occurs when there are electrolyte and fluid imbalance that happens when malnourished people have been hospitalized for long and start eating again after long. Chances of getting refeeding syndrome increase when after not eating for over ten days and having a very low body weight. Thus, fasting is not recommended for underweight, poorly nourished, or deficient in any nutrients. This is the reason why carrying out a fast longer than a few days without medical supervision is not recommended. Multi-day fasting under five days without professional advice is all right, you should ensure that you eat nutritious meals. If you fast for longer, you should get customized support and supervision from a healthcare professional. This emphasizes the point of eating a nutritious diet when practicing intermittent fasting. Do not make fasting deteriorate your general well-being, take good care of yourself.

People who cannot Fast on the 8:16 Plan

Intermittent Fasting can work for anyone. It can help anyone get healthy, lose weight and build lean muscles. However, there are a few exceptions. These exceptions are mainly for safety and health reasons. There are certain current health conditions that may worsen when you enter long fasting periods.

Sleep deprived or stressed

People who are experiencing high-stress levels for quite a long time are not good candidates for long fasting periods. These also include those who are sleep-deprived. Sleep deprivation and chronic high stress levels take a huge toll on health. Add fasting periods and the body will be subjected to extremely high strain. This can seriously deplete the body's capability to compensate and keep the organs working, further leading to a host of serious, potentially fatal conditions. There can be accelerated cell aging and death, accumulation of toxins, reduced immunity and slowing of metabolism and organ functioning.

It is advisable to address stress and sleep deprivation first before going in the IF lifestyle.

Sugar or food addict

If you have an addiction to sugar or certain food, fasting will become especially difficult. You will experience intensified cravings. If you are trying to wean off sugar, then fasting may cause you to relapse. There is a huge possibility that you will gorge on high sugar foods during the eating window. It is better to find other ways to deal with sugar addiction.

Medication

The actions of certain medications are affected by conditions in the body. Adjustments in dosages may be necessary. If you are taking medications for any health condition, inform your doctor about your plan in following the IF diet. Discuss with your doctor first before jumping into the IF life.

Pregnant and breastfeeding women, children

These people have high nutritional requirements for various metabolic and growth needs. Pregnant women need to eat to provide for the nutritional needs of the baby. Prolonged fasting states in pregnant women can lead to weakness and some potential complications like poor fetal growth.

For breastfeeding women, long fasting periods are also not recommended. They need to eat because they have to retain a good supply of nutrients for breast milk production. They also need the energy to replenish what they lost during the milk production process and the breastfeeding sessions. This stage can be really taxing on a woman's strength.

Children are at a stage of rapid growth and development. They have high nutritional requirements to fuel growth spurt and the maturation of their various organs. This is not the time to force their bodies into relying on fat stores during fasted states. It is still better for children to eat nutritious foods whenever they are hungry.

Chapter 10:
Organic Or Non-Organic Food-What Should You Eat

When you hear organic, you surely know – minus synthetic fertilizers. You also appreciate it is minus pesticides. Again correct. Now, those are the two factors that distinguish organic foods from non-organic ones. But you realize that the farmer would need to disclose those facts to you otherwise you would not know how the food was grown. Still, the farmer might be gracious enough to disclose to a store owner the fact that the food is not organic, but the trader might decide to veil that fact behind some jargon.

Organic foods contain organic and not artificial materials. The set standards for these foods vary from one country to another but they must all follow whatever regulations are set.

Organic foods aren't strictly fruits and vegetables as many may tend to believe.

So, are there any physical signs that can tell you, as a consumer, that certain food is likely to be organic or not? Yes, luckily, there are. Like the innocent, genuine village folk, organic food may not have much cosmetic appeal, but it distinctly tastes great. A good example is the organic carrots that have a rugged look that could sometimes make you frown, but which are sweet in an irresistible way.

And on that note, you might wonder, why not try and change that rather rough look of many organic foods? Well, you do not want to go that way because it would be copying the growers of foods of that are not organic; those who use chemical material to wax their products smooth.

Here are attractive features of organic food:

- It is healthy. By eating organic, you drastically lower the chance of disease that is triggered by use of chemicals and other synthetic products on crops and animals. Such diseases include the dreaded cancer.

- Higher in nutrition. What does that mean, considering that there is no mention of the main nutrients – protein, carbohydrates and fats?

- It is not genetically modified. Antioxidants effectively clean your body cells, thus making your body not susceptible to disease. Just like a dirty floor draws pests, when your body is full of bad elements, otherwise referred to as free radicals, it is great ground for disease causing organisms. And those free radicals are the ones that get cleared by the antioxidants. So we are talking of organic foods helping to keep your hospital bills in check; and, of course, you being able to lead a healthy life.

Why You Need to Eat Organic Foods

As long as you realize that inorganic foods are an easy gateway to disease, you will want to go for organic. There are actually direct and indirect advantages of pursuing organic foods. If many of you eat organic, more and more farmers will be motivated to produce food organically. You will thereby enjoy:

- A cleaner environment. This is because organic farming uses organic pest control substances as opposed to artificial insecticides. As a result, you have clean water sources and green fodder for your animals. This, you need to appreciate, is not a scholarly report that needs detailed analysis. Right from where you are, if you and your immediate neighbors are into organic farming, you will rarely find your families needing medical attention.

- Reduced pollution. Having organic farming is a great way to keep away diseases that come about from environmental pollution. You do not breathe dangerous gases from artificial pesticides and herbicides. That, obviously, implies a healthier and more productive life for you and your family.

- Water and soil conservation. When you eat organic and farmers stick to organic farming, what happens to the soil texture is very positive because there are no chemicals that would destroy it. On the other hand, manure that is used in place of synthetic fertilizers help to enrich the soil organically, leaving it strong in nutrients and in texture. As a result, the soil retains water longer, and food supply becomes more reliable than otherwise.

- Improving financial position. Did you know that every time you save on cost, it is like you are actually earning more income? Think of the amount of money you save when you cut down on hospital visits. In fact, consider how much money you save just by cutting down on Over the Counter drugs that are so common when you have frequent wheezing from a polluted environment; or even irritated skin from the chemical triggered allergies. This is money that becomes available to improve your quality of life in other more pleasant ways.

- Food that is clear of artificial preservatives and also additives. You will be pleased to know that the organizations that are charged with the role of certifying organic foods also restrict the use of additives and artificial preservatives in packed foods. This is a way of ensuring that your naturally produced food is not interfered with at the last stages; maintaining the organic status of the food.

By choosing to eat organically, you can avoid a lot of GMO's and pesticides that are a normal part of our food. There are so many pesticides used that it is estimated that the average American consumes 16 pounds of pesticides a year through the food that they eat. Organic food is free of these pesticides. Organic food farmers use tried and true farming methods. They manage and nourish their soil, they don't use pesticides and they avoid GMO foods. Because of these basic farming practices, the food not only avoids the contamination of pesticides but it actually has more nutrients and even tastes better than non-organic food. It may be hard to switch to an organic lifestyle mainly because it is more expensive.

Your expense is justified in that you are spending more to help support a more sustainable lifestyle. In addition, you can cut the cost of your food by growing and eating your own food from your own garden.

Organic farmers used tried and true farming practices. These farming practices use nutrient-rich soil. By growing food in nutrient-rich soil, in turn, your food that you are consuming also is rich in nutrients. By eating organically, you not only avoid pesticides but you are eating a healthier product, which in turn will help your body get the vitamins and minerals it needs. By practicing your own organic farming methods, you can benefit from this healthier lifestyle.

Non-Organic foods

GMOs are not organic because really, farmers of GMOs really babysit them; spraying herbicides to protect them against fluctuating weather conditions, and such other chemical-related treatments that ensure a bumper harvest. How about those internal processes those ensure that a GMO tomato is smoother and glossier than a baby's cheek, and a carrot is as straight and smooth as nothing else could be? Are those not scientific processes that distort the organic make-up of the product? For sure, GMOs cannot pass the organic test.

Genetically Modified Organisms (or GMOs) have swept the world of consumption and biotechnology industry in a very controversial manner. The term itself has prompted several countries to ban their production. Many skeptical consumers have likewise challenged state laws in making GMO labeling mandatory in all food products sold on the market.

And not only will you be better advised to keep off GMOs, you will also be asked to be keen if farms in the neighborhood are growing GMOs. The reason is that a lot of cross-pollination takes place, mostly through the wind, and organic crops in the neighborhood are likely to be thus polluted.

In addition, the effect of strong pesticides is likely to also find its way to neighboring organic farms. So, when you go shopping, even as you read the label that indicates that the food is organic, have a look at its source. If you have more than one option, go for the option whose source is in a neighborhood famous for organic farms. Playing safe in matters of healthy eating is not arrogance; it is only being proactive in a bid to live a longer and healthier life.

In short, organic foods are foods you will not worry about even when you eat them raw; in any case, there is no evil within that you are trying to kill through fire. But with natural foods, we see nobody trying to vouch for them. If we are to eat them, we can only rely on hope. In fact, if you think of ordinary water, which in any case we deem natural, is it of any nutritional value to you? Of course it is not.

Water is good alright, because it helps you sweat out excess salts and do a few more things that make you comfortable, but it will not add any vitamins, proteins, and such other nutrients to your body. So, much as natural foods are not necessarily bad, they do not fall under the realm of foods whose benefits you can evaluate before sale.

Eating organic is not just for the rural folk to whom this kind of eating comes more or less naturally. It is something that has become the in-thing, particularly to those that are enlightened in matters of health. But, granted, organic eating did not begin as the first choice for the rich and famous – no. For many years, moneyed people ate a sophisticated diet that was dominated by processed non-organic foods. Then ailments emerged; and doctors became more and more concerned as they realized that some of the serious ailments emerging are as a result of inorganic diet. And thus came the wisdom of organic eating.

Difference Between Organic and Non-organic Foods?

The first one is that organic food is grown using natural fertilizer. The inorganic one is grown using synthetic fertilizers.

The second difference is that pest control is through natural means such as the use of birds, traps, insects, or natural pesticides. On the other hand, the inorganic ones have pests controlled using synthetic fertilizers.

The third one that you should be conscious of is that animal products like eggs, milk and meat are free from GMOs and hormones. Livestock reared under inorganic conditions are fed hormones to grow faster.

Fighting diseases under organic involves zero-grazing, rotational grazing and so on. Under the non-organic, medications such as antibiotics are used.

Lastly, the livestock under the organic farming are enclosed or confined. On the other hand, the non-organic ones are free to roam.

This has ultimately made organic foods become one of the fastest growing sectors of the American Food Industry today.

Reasons to Say NO to non-organic food

- Allergic reaction and adverse immune responses. Mice which were fed with alpha-amylase inhibitor (insecticidal protein) sustained a strong immunity against GM protein. Antibodies were developed, which allowed the hypersensitivity reaction to delay. This means that the insecticidal protein acts as a sensitizer, which made the mice more susceptible to developing allergies as compared to consuming non-allergenic type of food.
- Presence of lesions in the stomach. Ulcers and stomach lesions developed in rats that were fed with GM tomatoes for a period of 28 days. More disturbingly, the study found unexplained deaths among 20% of the 40 rats used in the laboratory test. This particular study was commissioned by the company Calgene, the producer of the GMO tomato called Flavr Savr.
- Aging of the liver. Another experiment carried out utilized GM soy fed to mice for a period of 2 years. The result showed rapid changes in the hepatocyte metabolism. Moreover, indications of liver aging such as calcium signaling and stress response changes

were found. Mice, which were fed with non-GMO soy showed complete normal liver function.

- Dense uterine lining. For a period of 15 months, female rats were given genetically engineered soy. At the end of the test period, results show significant thickening in the lining of the uterus. Additionally, the study recorded changes in the ovaries of these mice as compared to those who took non-GMO soy. The lining of the uterus, also referred to as the epithelium, had higher number of cells.

- Unstable functioning of the pancreas, testes, and liver. The internal organs of mice fed with GMO soy demonstrated instability, particularly for the pancreas, testes, and liver. After tests were conducted, scientists have found that there was an abnormal formation of nuclei and nucleoli among the liver cells.

- Presence of toxins in the liver and kidney. There are now 19 different studies showing the effects of GMO soy and Bt Maize in mammals. Among the most disturbing results is the consistent and heavy presence of toxins in the liver and kidneys. Long-term feeding trials are currently under-way to validate the chronicity of this condition.

- Altered gut bacteria formation and blood biochemistry. Using GMO rice for 90 days, rats demonstrated an increased water intake. These GMO rice-fed rats displaced unstable blood biochemistry. Presence of altered bacteria in the gut was observed, which could consequently lead to disturbed digestive system functions and inefficient nutrition absorption.

- Enlarged liver. Monsanto GM canola was used in another study involving rats. For a period of four weeks, these rats developed enlarged organs, particularly the liver. Abnormal increase in the liver size is a sign of toxicity.

Chapter 11:
Breakfast
Eggs in A Hole

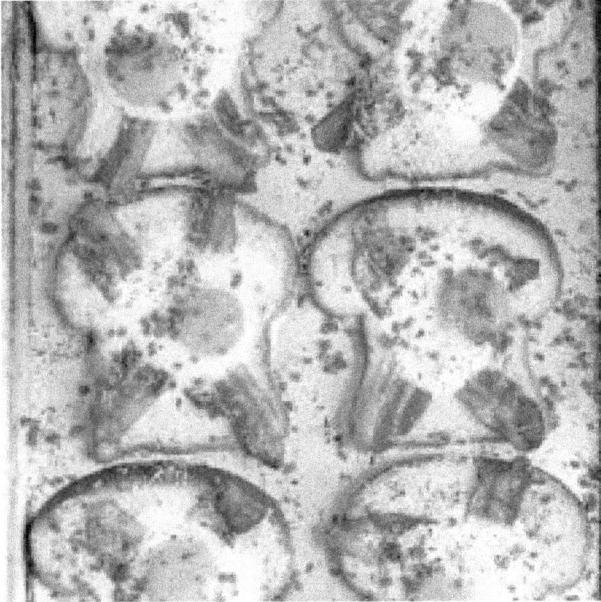

Serving: 2

Preparation Time: 10 minutes

Cooking Time: 1 0 minutes

 Ingredients

2 and ½ slices whole wheat bread

Olive oil spray

Fresh ground pepper

Hot sauce to taste

Salt to taste

2 and ½ ounces avocado flesh, mashed

2 large eggs

Directions

Take your bread slices and make a hole in the middle using a cookie cutter

Season avocado mash with salt and pepper

Take a skillet and place it over medium-low heat, grease with cooking spray

Place bread slices and a cut portion in the skillet

Break the egg into the hole of the bread, cook until the egg properly settles down, season with more salt and pepper

Flip and cook the other side

Once done, transfer to a plate

Top the egg with avocado mash, hot sauce and crumble bread (made from the cut piece)

Enjoy!

Nutrition:

Calories: 229

Fat: 23g

Carbohydrates: 10g

Protein: 12g

Tomato and Egg Scramble

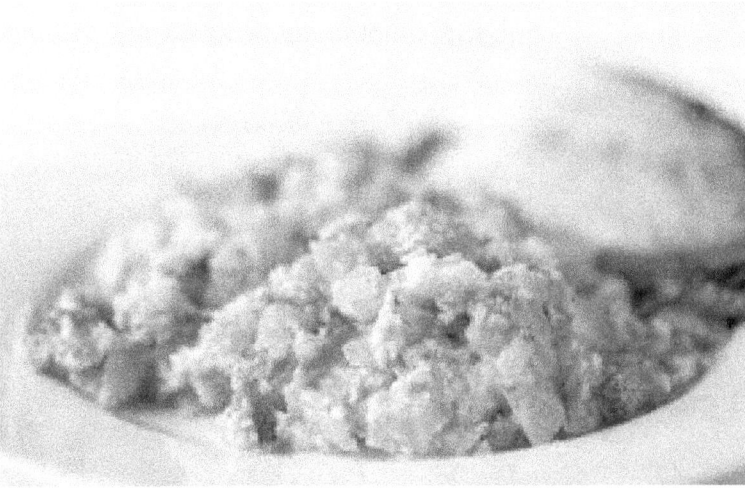

Serving: 2

Preparation Time: 10 minutes

Cooking Time: 5 minutes

Ingredients

8 whole eggs

½ cup fresh basil, chopped

2 tablespoons olive oil

½ teaspoon red pepper flakes, crushed

1 cup grape tomatoes, chopped

Salt and pepper to taste

Directions

Take a bowl and whisk in eggs, salt, pepper, red pepper flakes and mix well

Add tomatoes, basil, and mix

Take a skillet and place it over medium-high heat

Add egg mixture and cook for 5 minutes and cooked and scrambled

Enjoy!

Nutrition:

Calories: 130

Fat: 10g

Carbohydrates: 8g

Protein: 1.8g

Hearty Pancakes

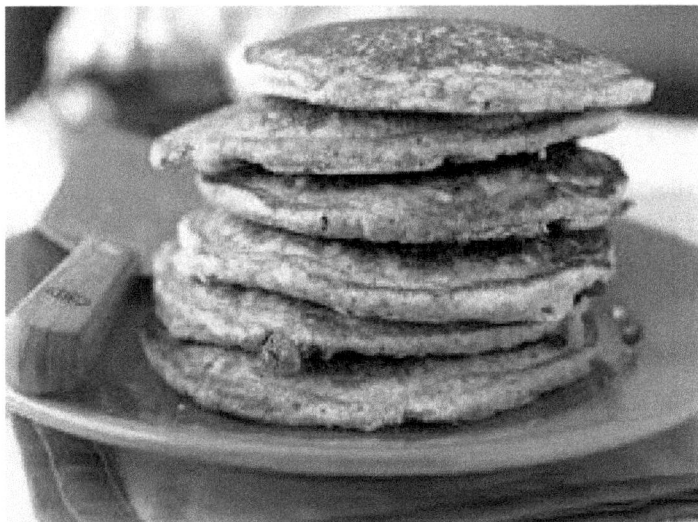

Serving: 4

Preparation Time: 10 minutes

Cooking Time: 5 minutes

Ingredients

1 teaspoon salt

½ cup low-fat milk

1 cup all-purpose flour

1 teaspoon vanilla

4 beaten eggs

1 teaspoon baking soda

2 cups non-fat Greek yogurt

Directions

Add Greek yogurt to your bowl and mix in the dry ingredients in another bowl

Stir the mixture into your yogurt and make sure everything is mixed well

Stir in eggs, milk, vanilla and stir well

Stir the mixture into the yogurt batter and add more flour to thicken it up

Take a skillet and place it over medium heat, add pancake batter and cook until bubbles appear

Flip and cook the other side

Nutrition:

Calorie: 212

Fat: 2g

Carbohydrates: 28g

Protein: 2g

Pineapple Oatmeal

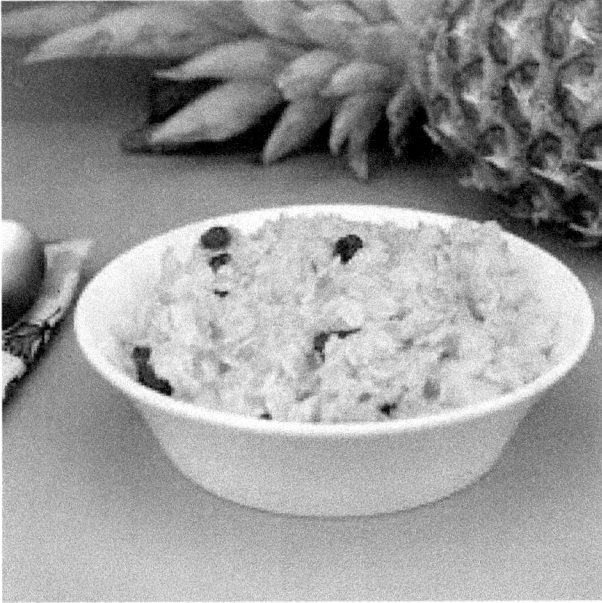

Serving: 5

Preparation Time: 10 minutes

Cooking Time: 4-8 hours

 Ingredients

1 cup steel-cut oats

4 cups unsweetened almond milk

2 medium apples, slashed

1 teaspoon coconut oil

1 teaspoon cinnamon

¼ teaspoon nutmeg

2 tablespoons maple syrup

A drizzle of lemon juice

Directions

Add listed ingredients to a cooking pan and mix well

Cook on very low flame for 8 hours/ or on high flame for 4 hours

Gently stir

Add toppings your desired toppings

Serve and enjoy!

Store in the fridge for later use, make sure to add a splash of almond milk after reheating for added flavor

Nutrition:

Calories: 180

Fat: 5g

Carbohydrates: 31g

Protein: 5g

Delicious Pumpkin Pie Oatmeal

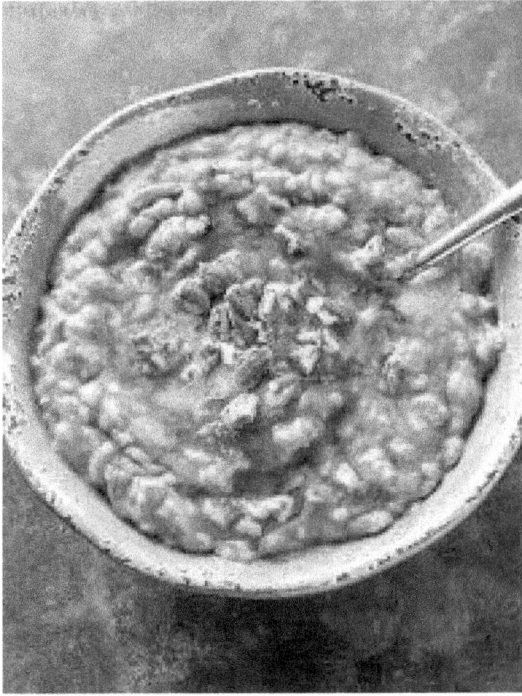

Serving: 2

Preparation Time: 10 minutes

Cooking Time: 10 minutes

Servings: 4

 Ingredients

½ cup canned pumpkin

Mashed banana as needed

¾ cup unsweetened almond milk

½ teaspoon pumpkin pie spice

1 cup oats

2 teaspoons maple syrup

Directions

Mash banana using fork and mix in the remaining ingredients (except oats) and mix well

Add oats and finely stir

Transfer mixture to a pot and let the oats cook until it has absorbed the liquid and are tender

Serve and enjoy!

Nutrition:

Calories: 264

Fat: 4g

Carbohydrates: 52g

Protein: 7g

Egg Muffins

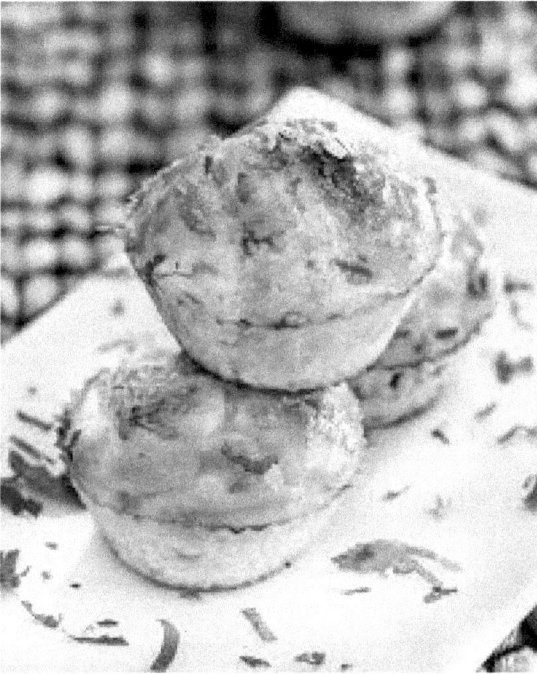

Serving: 6

Preparation Time: 10 minutes

Cooking Time: 30 minutes

Servings: 4

 Ingredients

½ teaspoon sage

½ teaspoon pepper

¼ teaspoon red pepper flakes

½ pound ground turkey

1 bell pepper, diced

12 whole eggs

¼ teaspoon salt

¼ teaspoon Marjoram

Directions

Preheat your oven to 350 degrees F

Grease a cupcake tin with non-stick spray

Take a skillet and place it over medium heat, add turkey and cook

Beat in eggs with seasoning, stir in bell pepper and cooked turkey to the egg mixture

Divide egg mixture between muffin tins and bake for 30 minutes

Once the eggs are set, enjoy!

Nutrition:

Calories: 172

Fat: 10g

Carbohydrates: 2g

Protein: 16g

Avocado Breakfast

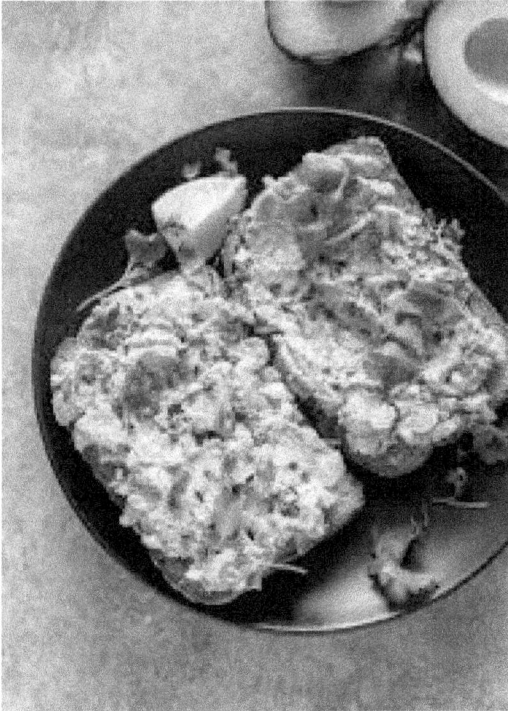

Preparation Time: 10 minutes

Cooking Time: 30 minutes

Servings: 4

Ingredients

2 whole grain tortillas (6 inch diameter)

2 eggs

2 tsp olive oil

1 avocado, peeled and seeded

1 tsp lemon juice

salt and pepper, to taste

Directions

First, warm tortillas in the microwave for approximately 30 seconds. Set aside.

In a small bowl, combine the avocado and lemon juice. Mix well until the mixture has a smooth consistency. Season with salt and pepper to taste.

Spread avocado mixture in an even layer on both tortillas. Set aside.

Heat a skillet greased with the olive oil at medium heat until just hot enough to sizzle a drop of water.

Break eggs and gently add to the skillet. Immediately reduce heat to low.

Place warm eggs on top of the tortillas and season with salt and pepper as desired.

Superfood Smoothie

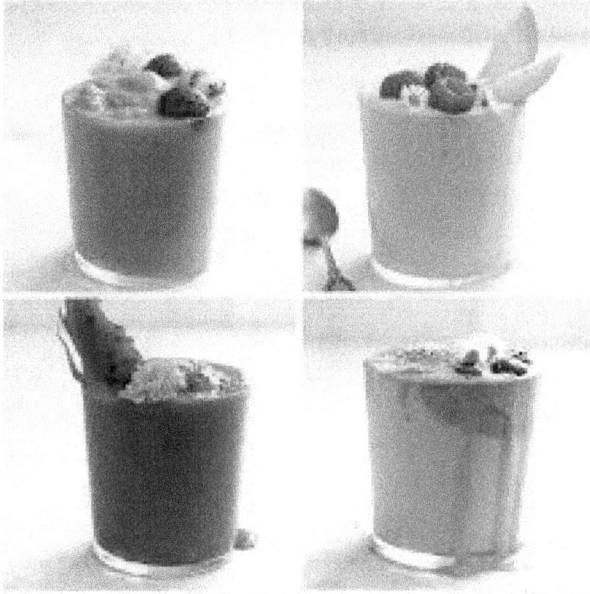

Preparation Time: 10 minutes

Cooking Time: 30 minutes

Ingredients

1 organic (sweet) apple, cored, keep peeling

1 cup frozen red grapes

1 teaspoon freshly grated ginger

1/2 cup kefir, plain, fat free

1/2 cup chilled green tea, unsweetened, home brewed is best

Directions

Chapter 12:
Lunch
Scallops and Jalapeno Vinaigrette

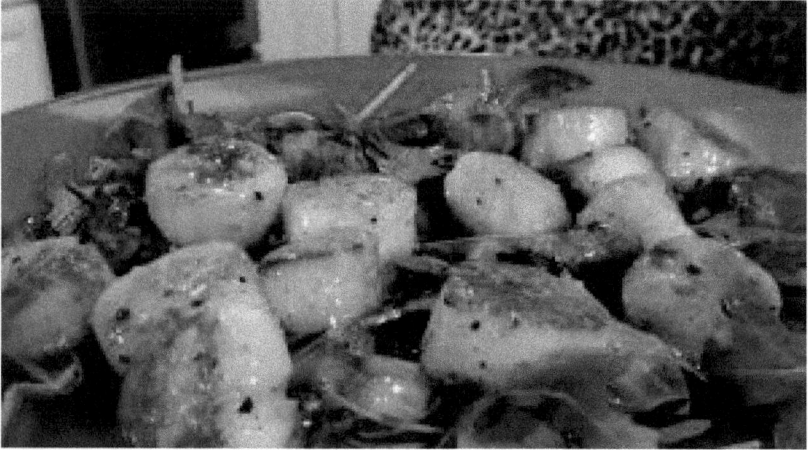

Preparation time: 5 minutes

Cooking time: 6 minutes

Servings: 4

Ingredients:

1 jalapeno pepper, seedless and minced

¼ cup extra virgin olive oil

¼ cup rice vinegar

¼ teaspoon mustard

Black pepper to the taste

A pinch cayenne pepper

1 tablespoon vegetable oil

12 big sea scallops

2 oranges, sliced

Directions:

In your blender, mix jalapeno with olive oil, mustard, black and vinegar and pulse really well.

Season scallops with cayenne pepper.

Heat up a pan with the vegetable oil over high temperature, add scallops and cook them for 3 minutes on each side.

Divide scallops on plates, place orange slices on top and drizzle the jalapeno vinaigrette.

Coconut Lobster Tails

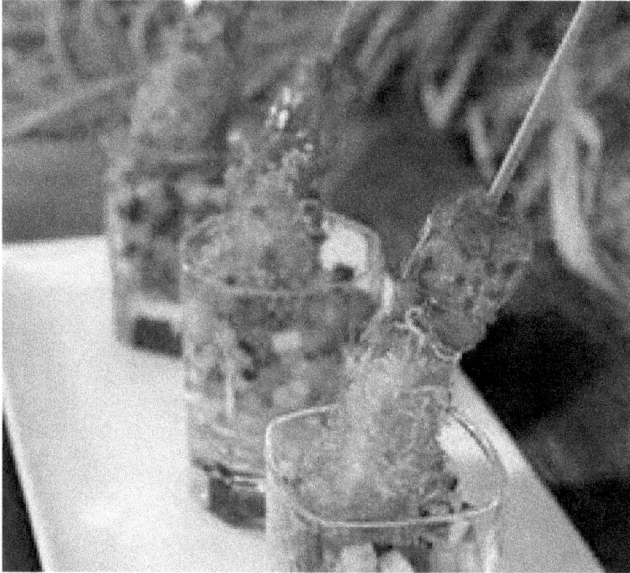

Preparation time:10 minutes

Cooking time: 10 minutes

 Servings: 2

Ingredients:

2 big whole lobster tails

½ teaspoon paprika

½ cup coconut butter

White pepper to the taste

1 lemon cut in wedges

Directions

Place lobster tails on a baking sheet, cut top side of lobster shells and pull them apart

Season with white pepper and paprika.

Add butter and toss gently

Introduce lobster tails in preheated broiler and broil for 10 minutes.

Divide on plates, garnish with lemon wedges and serve right away!

Nutrition value per

Serving: Calories 140, fat 2, fiber 2, carbs 6, protein 6

Tuna and Orange Salsa

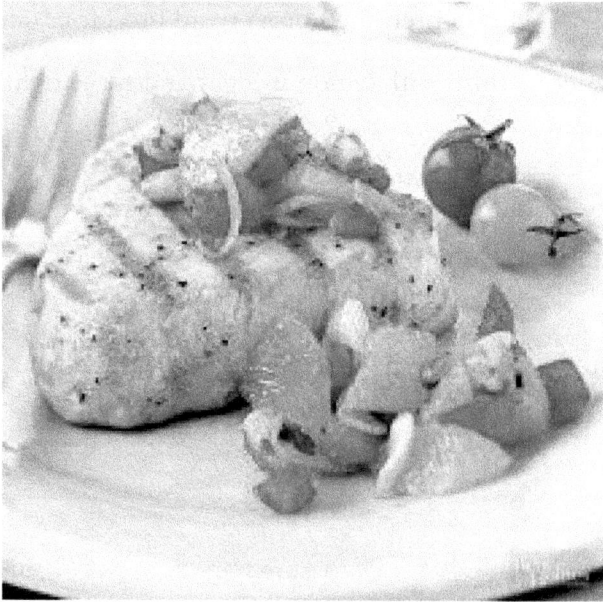

Preparation time:10 minutes

Cooking time: 5 minutes

 Servings: 4

Ingredients:

2 oranges, sliced

½ cup red onion, chopped

1 red bell pepper, chopped

¼ cup mint, chopped

1 tablespoon red wine vinegar

1 tablespoon vegetable oil

Black pepper to the taste

4 tuna steaks

1 teaspoon coriander, dried

Directions:

In a bowl, mix oranges with onion, bell pepper, mint, vinegar, salt and pepper, stir and leave aside for now.

Heat up your kitchen grill over medium high heat, rub tuna steaks with oil, pepper and coriander and grill for about 5 minutes.

Divide on plates, top with the orange salsa you've prepared and serve.

Nutrition value per

Serving: Calories 140, fat 2, fiber 3, carbs 9, protein 4

Parsley Seafood Stew

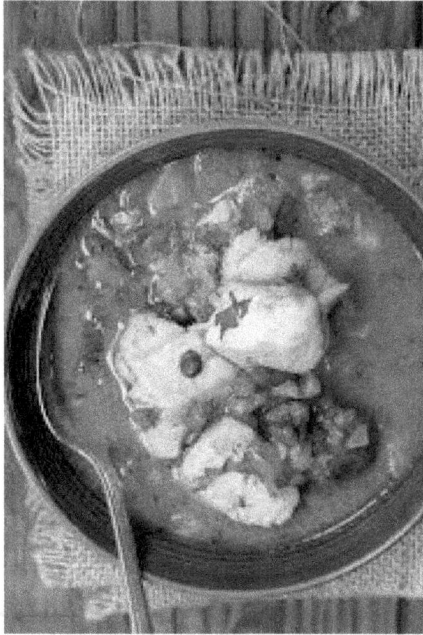

Preparation time:10 minutes

Cooking time: 12 minutes

Servings: 4

Ingredients:

12 jumbo shrimp, peeled (shells reserved) and deveined

4 parsley springs

¼ cup parsley, chopped

1 garlic clove, minced

1 tablespoon garlic, minced

1 tablespoon extra virgin olive oil

¼ cup shallot, chopped

1 cup dry white wine

2 dozen clams, scrubbed

1 pound mussels, scrubbed

Black pepper to the taste

1 tomato, chopped

8 scallops halved horizontally

2 cups water

Directions:

Heat up a pan over high heat, add shrimp shells and 1 garlic clove, stir and cook for 2 minutes.

Add parsley springs and water, stir, bring to a boil, cook for 3 minutes, strain into a bowl and leave aside for now.

Meanwhile, heat up another pan with the olive oil over medium high heat, add 1 tablespoon garlic and shallots, stir and cook for 1 minute.

Add wine and shrimp stock, add clams and mussels, bring to a simmer and cook for 4 minutes until clams open.

Divide clams and mussels into bowls, sprinkle chopped parsley and leave aside.

Season broth with black pepper, add scallops, shrimp and tomato, cover and cook for 2 more minutes over medium heat.

Add this mix to the bowls with the clams and mussels sprinkle chopped parsley and serve.

Nutrition value per

Serving: Calories 150, fat 2, fiber 3, carbs 7, protein 3

Bacon and Chicken Garlic Wrap

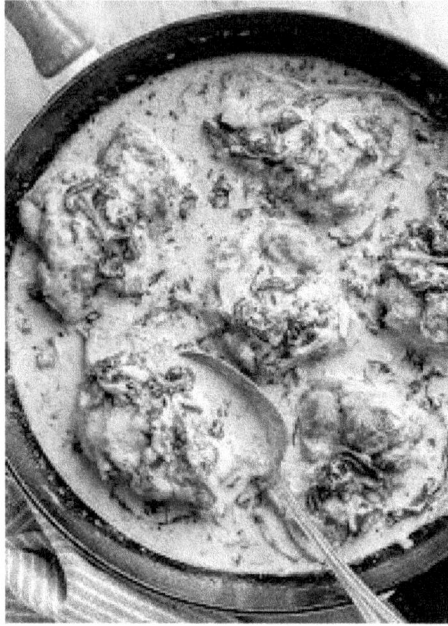

Serving: 4

Preparation Time: 15 minutes

Cooking Time: 10 minutes

 Ingredients

1 chicken fillet, cut into small cubes

8-9 thin slices bacon, cut to fit cubes

6 garlic cloves, minced

How To

Preheat your oven to 400 degrees F

Line a baking tray with aluminum foil

Add minced garlic to a bowl and rub each chicken piece with it

Wrap bacon piece around each garlic chicken bite

Secure with toothpick

Transfer bites to the baking sheet, keeping a little bit of space between them

Bake for about 15-20 minutes until crispy

Serve and enjoy!

Nutrition (Per Serving)

Calories: 260

Fat: 19g

Carbohydrates: 5g

Protein: 22g

Blackened Chicken

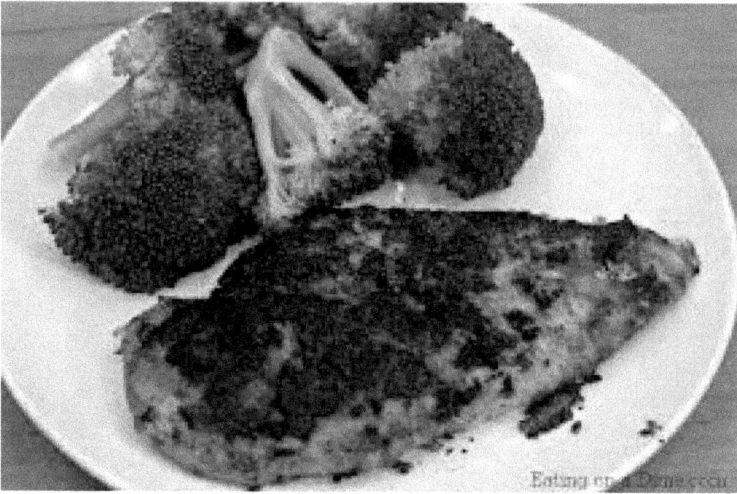

Serving: 4

Preparation Time: 10 minutes

Cooking Time: 10 minutes Ingredients

½ teaspoon papri ka

1/8 teaspoon salt

¼ teaspoon cayenne pepper

¼ teaspoon ground cumin

¼ teaspoon dried thyme

1/8 teaspoon ground white pepper

1/8 teaspoon onion powder

2 chicken breasts, boneless and skinless

Directions

Preheat your oven to 350 degrees Fahrenheit

Grease baking sheet

Take a cast-iron skillet and place it over high heat

Add oil and heat it up for 5 minutes until smoking hot

Take a small bowl and mix salt, paprika, cumin, white pepper, cayenne, thyme, onion powder

Oil the chicken breast on both sides and coat the breast with the spice mix

Transfer to your hot pan and cook for 1 minute per side

Transfer to your prepared baking sheet and bake for 5 minutes

Serve and enjoy!

Nutrition (Per Serving)

Calories: 136

Fat: 3g

Carbohydrates: 1g

Protein: 24g

Clean Parsley and Chicken Breast

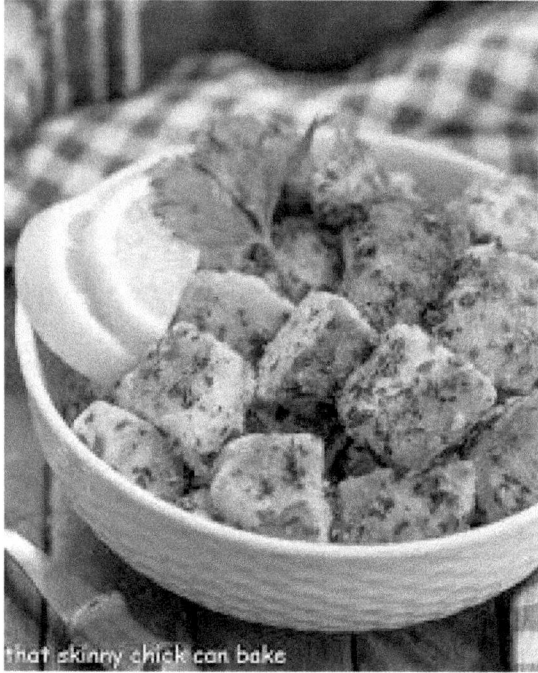

that skinny chick can bake

Serving: 4

Preparation Time: 10 minutes

Cooking Time: 40 minutes

 Ingredients

1 tablespoon dry parsley

1 tablespoon dry basil

4 chicken breast halves, boneless and skinless

½ teaspoon salt

½ teaspoon red pepper flakes, crushed

2 tomatoes, sliced

How To

Preheat your oven to 350 degrees F

Take a 9x13 inch baking dish and grease it up with cooking spray

Sprinkle 1 tablespoon of parsley, 1 teaspoon of basil and spread the mixture over your baking dish

Arrange the chicken breast halves over the dish and sprinkle garlic slices on top

Take a small bowl and add 1 teaspoon parsley, 1 teaspoon of basil, salt, basil, red pepper and mix well. Pour the mixture over the chicken breast

Top with tomato slices and cover, bake for 25 minutes

Remove the cover and bake for 15 minutes more

Serve and enjoy!

Nutrition (Per Serving)

Calories: 150

Fat: 4g

Carbohydrates: 4g

Protein: 25g

Chapter 13:
Dinner
White Steamed Fish

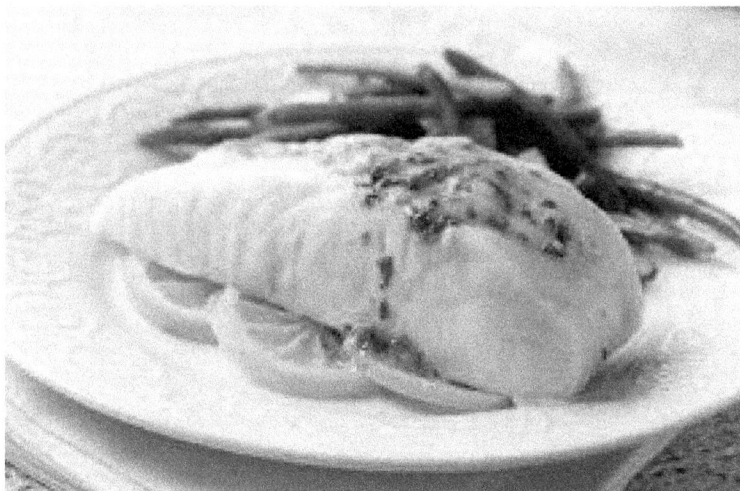

Preparation time: 10 minutes

Cooking time: 10 minutes

Servings: 4

Ingredients:

4 white fish fillets

1 tablespoon olive oil

1 teaspoon thyme, dried

1 pound cherry tomatoes, halved

1 cup black olives, pitted and chopped, soaked for 5 hours

A pinch of sea salt and black pepper

1 garlic clove, minced

1 cup water

Directions:

Put the water in your instant pot, place the steamer basket on top and arrange fish inside.

Season with salt, pepper, thyme and garlic.

Add oil, olives and tomatoes, rub gently, cover your instant pot and cook on Low for 10 minutes.

Release the pressure fast, divide fish and all veggies between plates and serve hot.

Nutrition value per

Serving: Calories 140, fat 2, fiber 2, carbs 8, protein 2

Shrimp Umani

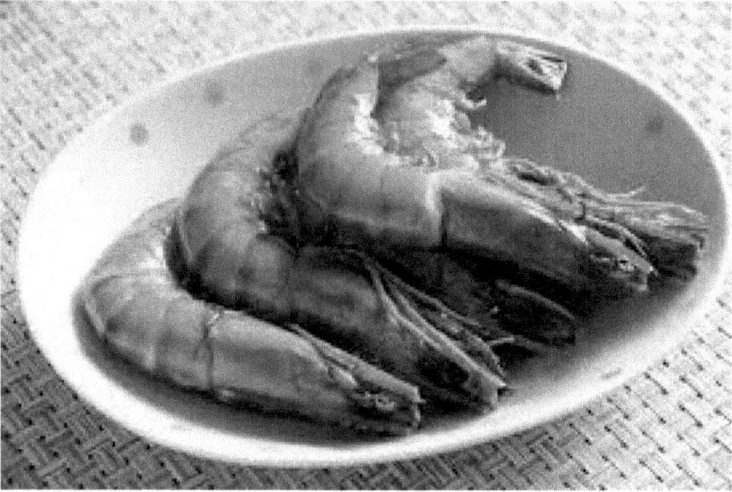

Preparation time: 10 minutes

Cooking time:3 minutes

 Servings: 2

Ingredients:

8 big shrimp

1 tablespoon ginger, grated

3 tablespoons low sodium soy sauce

1/3 cup sake

1 cup dashi

3 tablespoons mirin

1 tablespoon sugar

Directions:

Heat up a pan with the dashi over medium heat, add sugar, ginger, soy sauce, mirin and sake, stir and bring to a boil.

Add shrimp, cook for 3 minutes, take off heat, leave aside to cool down completely, divide between 2 plates and serve.

Nutrition value per

Serving: Calories 100, fat 1, fiber 3, carbs 6, protein 3

Sake Herring Roe

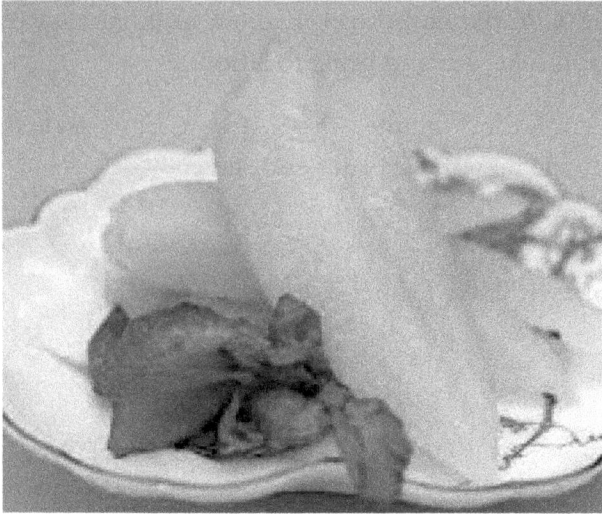

Preparation time: 10 minutes

Cooking time: 5 minutes

Servings: 4

Ingredients:

10 pieces herring roe, soaked in water for half a day and drained

3 cups water

Kombu, thinly sliced

3 tablespoons mirin

3 tablespoons sake

6 tablespoons low sodium soy sauce

1 teaspoon sugar

1 handful bonito flakes

Directions:

In a pot, mix water with kombu, mirin, sake, soy sauce and sugar, stir and bring to a boil over medium heat.

Add herring roe, cook for 2 minutes, take off heat and add bonito flakes.

Leave everything to cool down in the pot, divide herring roe into bowls and serve.

Nutrition value per

Serving: Calories 140, fat 2, fiber 3, carbs 6, protein 3

Mexican Shrimp Salad

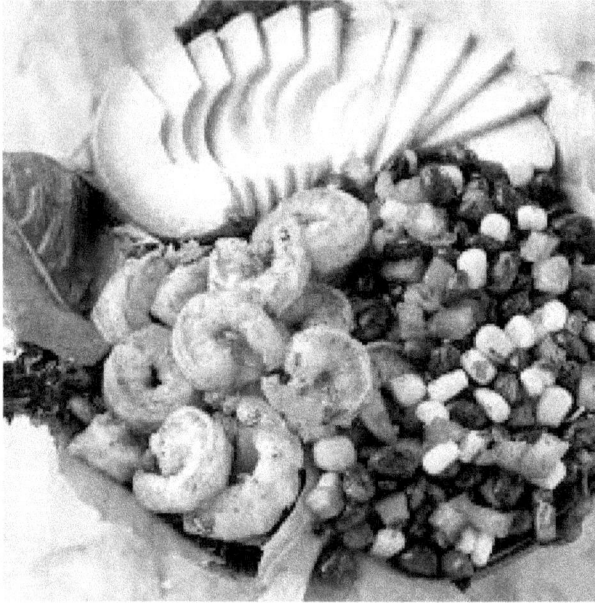

Preparation time: 10 minutes

Cooking time: 20 minutes

 Servings: 6

Ingredients:

1 pound shrimp, deveined and peeled

2 cups cherry tomatoes, halved

2 romaine lettuce hearts, shredded

1 cucumber, chopped

1 avocado, pitted, peeled and chopped

½ cup cilantro leaves, chopped

Black pepper to the taste

4 cups tortilla chips

2 tablespoons low fat sour cream

2 tablespoons lime juice

½ teaspoon lime zest, grated

Directions:

Put water in a pot, bring to a boil over medium high heat, add shrimp, cook for 3 minutes, transfer them to a bowl filled with ice water, drain, pat dry them and put in a salad bowl.

Add lettuce, cucumber, tomatoes, avocado, cilantro and tortilla chips.

In a bowl, mix sour cream with lime juice, lime zest, and black pepper to the taste and whisk well.

Pour this over salad, toss to coat and serve right away.

Nutrition value per

Serving: Calories 150, fat 2, fiber 4, carbs 7, protein 3

Ginger Tuna Kabobs

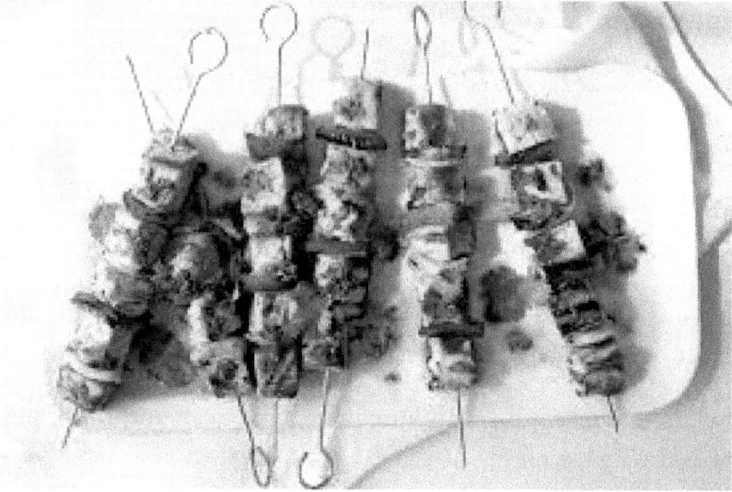

Preparation time: 30 minutes

Cooking time: 10 minutes

Servings: 16

Ingredients:

¼ cup low sodium soy sauce

1 pound tuna steaks, cubed in 16 pieces

2 tablespoons rice vinegar

Black pepper to the taste

1 tablespoon sesame seeds

2 tablespoons canola oil

16 pieces pickled ginger

1 bunch watercress

Directions:

In a bowl, mix soy sauce with vinegar and tuna, toss to coat, cover bowl and keep in the fridge for 30 minutes.

Discard marinade, pat dry tuna and sprinkle it with black pepper and sesame seeds.

Heat up a pan with the oil over medium heat, add tuna pieces, cook them until they are pink in the center and browned on the outside, take them off heat and transfer them to a plate.

Thread one ginger slice on 16 skewers.

Thread one tuna cube on each of the 16 skewers.

Arrange watercress on a platter, arrange tuna kabobs on top and serve.

Nutrition value per

Serving: Calories 150, fat 1, fiber 4, carbs 19, protein 4

Roasted Salmon

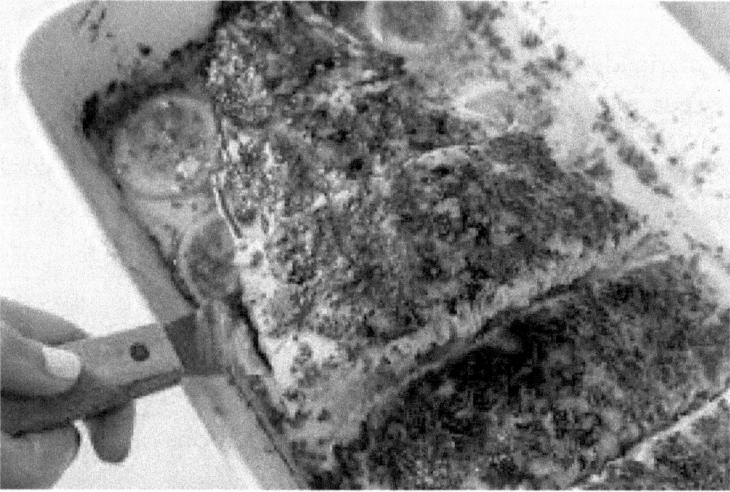

Preparation time: 10 minutes

Cooking time: 35 minutes

Servings: 6

Ingredients:

2 pounds salmon fil lets, boneless

1 garlic clove, minced

¼ cup maple syrup

¼ cup balsamic vinegar

A pinch of black pepper

Chopped mint for serving

Cooking spray

Directions:

Heat up a pan over medium low heat, add maple syrup, vinegar and garlic, stir and heat up for 1 minutes.

Transfer this to a bowl and leave aside to cool down a bit.

Spray a baking sheet with cooking spray, arrange salmon fillets on the sheet, season them with a pinch of black pepper and brush with half of the maple glaze.

Introduce in the oven at 450 degrees F and bake for 10 minutes.

Brush salmon with the rest of the glaze and bake for 20 minutes more.

Divide on plates, sprinkle mint on top and serve.

Nutrition value per

Serving: Calories 180, fat 2, fiber 4, carbs 10, protein 4

Lamb Meatballs and Mint Sauce

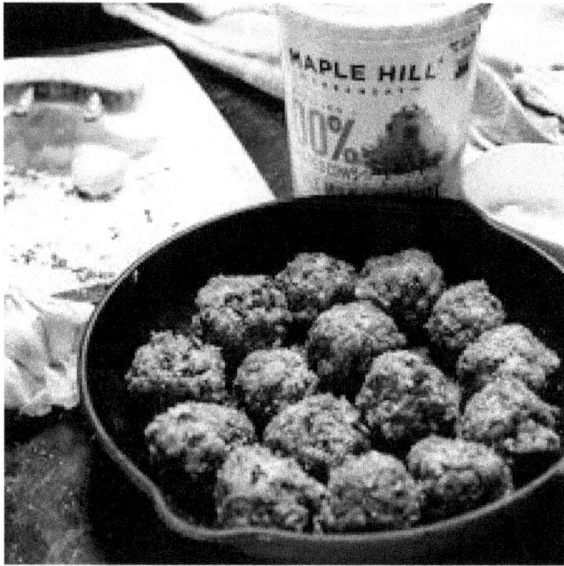

Preparation time: 10 minutes

Cooking time: 15 minutes

Servings:24

Ingredients:

10 ounces lamb meat, ground

2 teaspoons garlic, minced

2 teaspoons ginger, grated

2 teaspoons chili peppers, minced

2 tablespoons coriander, chopped

2 tablespoons low sodium fish sauce

1 egg

1 cup breadcrumbs

Black pepper to the taste

Vegetable oil for frying

2 tablespoons honey

For the mint sauce:

1 teaspoon ginger, grated

4 tablespoons rice wine

2 tablespoons low sodium soy sauce

2 tablespoons mint, chopped

1 teaspoon sugar

Back pepper to the taste

Directions:

In a bowl, mix lamb meat with 2 teaspoons ginger, garlic, chili, coriander, fish sauce, egg,black pepper to the taste and breadcrumbs and stir well.

Shape meatballs out of this mix and place them all on a working surface.

Heat up a large pan with the oil over medium high heat, add meatballs and cook them for 4 minutes on each side.

Transfer to paper towels, drain grease, drizzle the honey over them and arrange on a platter.

Meanwhile, in a bowl, mix 1 teaspoon ginger with rice vinegar, soy sauce, chopped mint, sugar and pepper to the taste.

Transfer sauce to small bowlsserve with your lamb meatballs.

Nutrition value per

Serving: Calories 279, fat 2, fiber 4, carbs 10, protein 10

Chapter 15:
7-day 16/8 intermittent fasting meal plan

DAY	BREAKFAST	LUNCH	DINNER
1.	Eggs in A Hole	Scallops and Jalapeno Vinaigrette	White Steamed Fish
2.	Tomato and Egg Scramble	Coconut Lobster Tails	Shrimp Umani
3.	Hearty Pancakes	Tuna and Orange Salsa	Sake Herring Roe
4.	Pineapple Oatmeal	Parsley Seafood Stew	Mexican Shrimp Salad
5.	Egg Muffins	Bacon and Chicken Garlic Wrap	Ginger Tuna Kabobs
6.	Avocado Breakfast	Blackened Chicken	Roasted Salmon
7.	Superfood Smoothie	Clean Parsley and Chicken Breast	Lamb Meatballs and Mint Sauce

Conclusion

Many people struggle with dieting plans and getting one that's capable of providing the desired results has always been a challenge. One thing that makes Intermittent fasting to be significant is the fact that fasting is a practice that comes so naturally to the body. It's easy to start fasting and flexible to sustain as you don't have to worry about the foods that you eat and the macronutrients.

I know that you have found valuable information regarding what 16:8 Intermittent fasting entails and how you can make use of it for optimal health and weight loss. Intermittent fasting doesn't have to be a struggle if you choose the right fasting protocol that suits you best and goes by the guidelines.

It's important to note that intermittent fasting is not a quick fix; you will not automatically lose weight just because you are fasting. You also have to watch your diet and ensure that the foods that you consume are helping you towards realizing your desired goal.

The path to a successful program of fasting can be quite difficult. Here are some rules for navigating the domain. Take it one step at a moment to comprehend the program's implications. Gradually try the fasting program. You do not just want to jump to something that might not be intended for you first. You can begin fasting once every three weeks before you adjust the time limit is gradually reduced as you wish. No one program operates the same manner for everyone. Choose a scheme and tailor it to your liking.

Decide if it is right for you. Even though there are some good benefits, remember IF is not for everyone. Your nutritional understanding and lifestyle exercise should determine if you are attempting IF. I strongly recommend that you first understand the essentials if you are new to exercise and nutrition. Begin with slowly, simply and gradually. There is no rush if you decide you would like to try IF. Choose one little thing to try, even if it is just a one-hour regular meal adjustment. Try this and see how it is working for you. Concentrate on what IF approaches have in common, rather than getting too into detail. Sometimes you eat and sometimes you do not do it that almost summarizes it.

Consider what is going on in your lives. Think about how much training you are doing and how intensively you are doing, how well you are resting and recovering, how well IF fits into your daily practice and ordinary personal operations; and what other pressure needs, and life provide. Remember IF one of the many types of diet is that function. But it "works" only when it is constant, flexible, and parts of your normal practice, not a duty, and not a permanent trigger of physical and psychological stress.

Know yourself and observe your experiences carefully. Be an academic and start gathering data, gaining knowledge, and drawing conclusions that you use to guide future action. Do the right thing for you. You should also give yourself time. Especially since it usually takes a few weeks to adapt to your new program. Difficulties are expected it is part of how life goes. It is life's element, they happen. You will figure out how to get more "ups" by staying open-minded and not panicking during the "downs." Think about what I want from IF. Focus on the process quality, not the outcome. IF is a great way to go psychologically

You need to be keenly conscious of how your body is responding to an ongoing program of fasting. Your body system will determine what you consume, how much time you consume, how much time you practice, how much calories you consume, etc. Considering all these variables will guarantee that you are in command of the program of fasting and eventually your weight.

You do not want to be in a rush watching your fat fly off your bones. Many of us are quite impatient with dumping one feeding regimen after another, as it does not work quickly enough. You need to realize that weight loss should be slow and for health reasons. It is okay to lose at most 2 pounds a week. Engage in your day-to-day operations while fasting as this is a time-flying route. Being idle will certainly hold your mind centered on meals, and here you can only imagine the result.

The most important advice is that you do not always have to consume. Just like in life, there is a moment for all we have set a timetable for. Therefore, the same applies to your pattern of eating. Fasting is not ironclad, working around it and setting up a program that operates for you is possible.